life on the
ground floor

LETTERS FROM THE EDGE OF EMERGENCY MEDICINE

life on the
ground floor

LETTERS FROM THE EDGE OF EMERGENCY MEDICINE

JAMES MASKALYK, M.D.

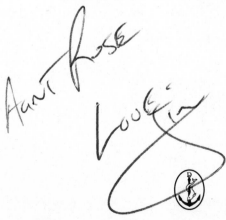

Doubleday Canada and colophon are registered trademarks of Penguin Random House Canada Limited

Library and Archives Canada Cataloguing in Publication

Maskalyk, James, 1973-, author
    Life on the ground floor / James Maskalyk.

Issued in print and electronic formats.
ISBN 978-0-385-66597-1 (hardback).—ISBN 978-0-385-67403-4 (epub)

    1. Emergency physicians. 2. Hospitals—Emergency services.
3. Emergency medicine. I. Title.

RA975.5.E5M38 2017   362.18   C2016-903009-1
                                            C2016-903010-5

Abiy Eshete courtesy of Makush Gallery
Printed and bound in the USA

Published in Canada by Doubleday Canada,
a division of Penguin Random House Canada Limited

www.penguinrandomhouse.ca

10 9 8 7 6 5 4 3 2 1

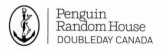

Penguin
Random House
DOUBLEDAY CANADA

TO MICHAEL.

Between stimulus and response, there is a space.

VIKTOR FRANKL

I'm at a friend's cottage, my toes creeping off the end of his dock. It is early summer 2007, and the water is grey and cold, like the sky. I am planning to dive in, and my balls are creeping as close as they can to my pelvis. Brr. I shiver. My phone buzzes beside my crumpled clothes. I reach down and pick it up, hoping for a long conversation. It is the university director of Toronto's emergency departments.

"James, it's Michael. Welcome back from Sudan. I've heard about some work in Ethiopia."

Say no, say no, say no, repeats inside my head, then, *It's next to Sudan.*

The wind blows harder.

"James?"

I step off the plane, queue for customs officers, Ethiopian visa in hand. A man holds a handwritten sign: "Dr. James—Toronto." Outside, the sun hurts my eyes and the air smells like home.

Aklilu leads me through a tin room, people on the floor. A few students lean against a wall. There is no nurse at triage.

"Next year, we are ready to begin."

Biruk and Sofia in the learning centre's wan light, feeling up and down each others' throats, learning where to cut if someone can't get a breath. Nazanin and Cheryl stand near, nodding or moving the students' fingers.

"Yes. Right there. Perfect."

I land back in Toronto's downtown emergency room. A man with his pant legs pulled to his knees, his feet black with frostbite from sleeping in the snow. A woman rolls on a stretcher, wiggling in pain. A doctor steps from a patient's room, holding a clear vial of spinal fluid to the light.

Crushed between cities, days mix with nights, and I can find little time to reflect or to write. My grandmother dies. My grandfather is alone.

I move to northern Alberta, and am at his kitchen table, looking out the window.

Snow blows sideways, and the woods are barely visible through the white static. The empty red hummingbird feeder swings from its hook. Past it, a squirrel jumps between branches of the pin cherry tree, and a cloud of white floats to the ground.

Cards shuffle in the next room, then a clack as he straightens the deck. He is playing solitaire. The furnace rumbles on, and a rush of warm air pours across the back of my neck. His game is lost in the sound.

He turned ninety this year, celebrated his sixty-seventh wedding anniversary, then mourned the death of his wife. I've come to his house by the lake, where he is struggling to remain as his body falls away. I've come here to care for him, and to learn from him, about how to be at the end of your life, having buried a wife and a son, because he's the wisest person I know.

I've come to write about emergency medicine, the "why" of it, and if the principles behind our striving to give a stranger's body another minute, another day, another year, are natural ones, why does it look so different in Addis and Toronto?

Yesterday, my grandfather and I drove to the trapline he's had since such plots of land were first deeded, seventy years ago. We rumbled across cattle grates, turned from an empty gravel road to a cut-line, filled with snow. He wanted to check his small trapper's cabin, make sure the door hadn't been punched in by a bear, and look at his traps. He had set three. The first two were empty; the third held a fisher, an animal like a wolverine, its face crushed into a final grimace, hard from the cold. I threw it in the back of the truck with a clunk. He would skin it later.

You don't live so close to the land without understanding that one way or another, in a snare, on the wrong side of a gun, or wasting slowly in a hospital bed, the end is one thing you don't have to look for. It's on the way.

I find myself near the end often because I work in emergency rooms. All the ones I've seen are on the ground floor. It allows for the easiest flow of life through the curtained rooms, because for the sickest, sometimes a minute matters.

A month or two earlier, a student from Germany was in the ER to learn the type of medicine at work there. He found it uninspiring. During the first half of the shift, he saw only two patients, and despite it being busy I found him behind the nursing station, checking his email.

I tapped him on his shoulder and pointed to a person the paramedics were pushing past. She was frail, and arched into angles from lying on a bed she hadn't left in months. Her breathing was fast and shallow, her eyes closed. The paramedics took the orange blanket between them and lifted her, weightless as a balloon, into an empty bed. The nurses told me about her when she arrived at triage, no ventilator, no CPR. Comfort measures only.

"You see that lady in bed six?"

He nodded.

"I think she'll die soon," I said. "You ever seen that before?"

He shook his head.

"You should."

He looked away, put his phone back in his pocket. "I think I would rather see someone new," he said, took a chart from the pile, and walked towards a different bed.

I let him go. I should have encouraged him more. There was something I wanted him to see. Not just the changes in her body as her story drew to a close, how the heart tracing moved from fast and narrow to slow and wide, the breathing from shallow to ragged, hitched then stopped, so he might later recognize last gasps in a someone who wanted help. I wanted him to be there for the moment *after* her final half breath, when all the parts were still there—kidneys, brain, blood, gentle titrations of thyroid hormone, precise amounts of dissolved salt—but life was gone.

"What was that thing?" I would have asked.

I don't know, either, I would have said, but that's what you're here for. To help it, whatever it is.

Then I would have taught him what I know. Airway first, breathing next. Medicine is life caring for itself. To me, it's the greatest story.

"I'm no good for nothing," my grandfather said this morning, teetering on the edge of the car door, waving my hand away before taking a shaky step on the ice. That is his idea of worth, you see—to be of use.

It's quiet in here now. Just the whirring of the second hand from the clock behind me. No cards. I imagine he is watching the snow just like me, waiting. One doesn't become a good hunter without learning how to do that.

He doesn't talk much. I'm not sure when I'll ask him what it's like to be near the end of your life, but that's OK. He's already taught me. It's the same as any other time. You wake up in the morning, and take the day as it comes.

A is for airway.

From the moment we are pushed into the light, take a wet lungful of air, and scream out "How cold!" this body is ours alone, its beautiful eyes and grasping hands, and it is connected to the future by the airway.

If you run a finger from your lips past the soft underside of your chin, you'll feel a hard lump of bone halfway down your neck. This is your upper airway. This is what Biruk and Sofia were tracing. To me, it is the most important part of your body, because without an open one, there's no breathing, only trying.

When I was small, my grandfather showed me how to dangle small snares on a stick leaned on a tree, so squirrels would run into the loops. They struggled, the snare tightened, and with it, their tether to the breathing world. My brother and I would pick them up in the morning, stiff, dangling from their nooses.

You could skin them for fur, get a dollar or two. I never learned how to do it. Their bodies were small, and one nick through the hide would make them worthless. I would turn over in the bed of the one-room trapper's cabin, flip open my book.

My brother had patience. He sat in the middle of the floor on a wooden chair, squirrel on his lap, making the tiny cuts. The first ones took him twenty minutes, but he got faster. My grandfather sat beside him, knife flashing, then turned the skins inside out, stretched them on oval boards until they dried.

The airway isn't a real thing; its empty space over which a body pulls in wind as breath, then moves it out, vibrating it into cries and words, truths and lies. The hole there, at the vocal cords, is about the width of your smallest finger. I wonder how few of the thousand strangers we pass on the street know this secret, that their entire life depends on something so small? When it narrows, though, they know, and silent appeals begin.

Pleasepleasepleaseplease.

How do you know if that space has closed in a person? Have you seen a look of pure panic? Someone clutching their throat with eyes so wide they're lidless? An allergic woman who had eaten a peanut, sitting forward, all the cords on her neck stretched to squeak in another gasp but she couldn't make a sound, because that hole was swollen to nothing. I didn't need to hear her words to know what she was saying. Adrenalin sifted through her blood, made her hair stand on end, like a squirrel in a tightening wire.

Pleasepleasepleaseplease.

It's hard to kill a brightly living thing. More or less you must mean it. Someone who's on their way to dying, though, it's no trick at all. Make a mistake, or stand idly by. This early in the alphabet, they're the same thing.

This is important. If it's you who's tripped while chewing a piece of fruit, you will want to breathe in. Every part of you, down to your smallest cell.

Don't. That would be a mistake.

Breathe out.

Bend over.

Cough.

Pleasepleasepleaseplease.

Harder.

You have about three minutes before things start to close in. Add to your plea that someone nearby might notice, get you to a hospital with someone waiting who knows where to cut.

If it's you who notices the person, eyes wide, clawing at his throat, he'll be quiet, red, then blue. You'll join his panic; it just slips in like that. Though the feeling is mostly beyond your control, you don't need to act it out. Instead, move with purpose. It is panic's best antidote.

Give him the advice I gave you, shout it in his ear— "Cough!"—then clap him on the back. If he remains silent and frantic, move behind and circle his abdomen with your arms. Put one hand over your other fist, high on his belly, and jerk him firmly under the diaphragm, use his trapped half breath half scream to pop what's in the airway: out. If he's fallen, his fear fading with his oxygen, turn him on his back and push sharply on the same high part of his stomach. Try. Try. Try. Check his mouth in case something came out. You don't want it to fall back in.

Call an ambulance.

Try.

If he's as small as a baby, put him on your lap, face down, sloping away from you, and rap his back a few times. If that doesn't work, I don't know, I've never had this problem, I'm nervous now, and though I was never taught this, I think I would hoist him by his feet, right upside down, hold hard, not let go, hit his back, because it has been two minutes now. If gravity didn't drop it, I'd turn him on his back, push up on his small stomach. An ambulance best be on its way, if you are in a place that has those types of things, because even if he starts breathing again, he'll need a hospital. Small livers and lungs can be hurt by even little pushes.

Breathe.

Stopping a catastrophe from happening is more efficient than racing to fix one, though less exciting to write about. Still, if someone is asleep, dead drunk but uninjured, turn her on her side, up leg bent and forward to down leg, so if she coughs anything up, there will just be a mess to clean up in the morning, not a body. When you read of rock stars dying young in their sleep, it's often because they had no friend around to do this, and why you don't hear about it more often is that little is written about the lonely lives of alcoholics who don't write hits.

Sudden sicknesses have more dramatic cures. Sicknesses that grow slowly need more time and energy to tip the balance back, if they retreat at all. A shoulder knocked loose can be yanked back with a single pull, whereas one frozen stuck by arthritis may never fit back right. A chunk of apple in an airway can be freed with a smack on the back, but cancer may squeeze a throat so slowly that you don't appreciate it at all until you hear the rasping whistle of air moving through a tighter and tighter space.

Huuuhnnnhhhh-huuuuhhhhh-hunnnnnnhhhhhhh-huuuuhhhhh

That whistle is called stridor. You develop an ear for it.

When I arrived at the emergency room as a student for the first time, dozens of monitors beeped for attention. A patient retched, another cried in pain. "Move it!" a nurse shouted and pushed some kind of machine past. I was in a universe with no identifiable laws, so I made up its first: stay the hell out of the way.

With time, and immersion, I habituated to my new environment, and as it goes, accumulated responsibility. Now I'm scenery too, just part of the whirl. Of a burst of sounds that never ends, though, three stop me: 1) the overhead announcement, in case it asks for my urgent presence; 2) the deepening "bloop-bloooop-blooooooop" of a saturation monitor as the oxygen level in a patient's blood droops low; and 3) stridor, that angry low whistle of an airway closing, from cancer or infection or burns or a growing bruise in a woman cut from her belt, swinging in a prison cell.

The sound is a snoring, but pitched higher, more sinister. It is louder on inhalation, as tissue draws together from the negative pressure a diaphragm creates to draw in breath. This turbulence of a disappearing airway is among the most dangerous sounds in the world, and sometimes, the last one a person hears.

You don't hear it often, but you never forget the times you have. Last time was in Ethiopia A young man had fallen from a building and came to our tin ER with his head broken open and a mouth full of blood. His breath rasped.

Hear that? I asked one of the Ethiopian residents. It's the sound of a world collapsing.

If the airway won't stay open, there aren't many options. A rigid breathing tube, past the soft tongue and snoring back of the throat, to meet the hard rings of the trachea, will keep open the connection from inside to outside. Or if that hole's gone for good, too much cancer, too much blood and swelling, you must cut a mouth into the neck.

In medical school, I practised in classes, then in my dreams. Slowly moving closer to the living, I bent over a mannequin, squeaked a tube, rubber on rubber, into its perfect blind face, chemical fumes stinging my eyes. A year later, outside the operating room, I chatted with nervous people in the hallway who were waiting for surgery, stomachs growling. I watched their lips move, but didn't hear what they were saying, because they would soon be unconscious, and all that would matter was their airway. They breathed the gas, dropped to sleep, and the anaesthetist handed me tools from elbowing distance away, in case I started to lever on their upper teeth with the blade's metal handle, trying to see that pen-sized hole, but I didn't, I pulled away from them like she told me to, and the tube slid in like glass.

Then, the ER. Drunks with stomachs full of beer, beaten bloody on the street. Old ladies, last seen the night before at the top of the stairs. Burly men with beards stained nicotine brown too short of breath to sit still. Young Ethiopian men fallen five storeys onto a pile of eucalyptus sticks. From daydreams to live nightmares.

I don't care much for their words either, more their bodies. In a live person, placing the tube is not easy, so if he is not just about dead, it is easier if we make him that way, put him unconscious and poison his muscles with curare, so he lies still as a mannequin. This relaxes the neck enough for me to stick a flat blade past his tongue, pull his chin away hard and put the angled window of the vocal cords into view. He's paralyzed, so there's no gagging. No breathing either. That's the panicky part.

There are now about ninety seconds to put the tube into place before the oxygen starts to fall, and the process that's held it starts to unwind. Those moments are so perfectly drawn, they can seem full as hours, but a single "bloop-bloooop-blooooooop" and all the future wooshes into the past.

I was standing in the back, far away from the fallen man. There were many voices in the room. So many I couldn't pick out a single one. It was too loud. There was no saturation monitor.

A young doctor was at the patient's head, focused on the airway. He had given the patient curare. Ninety seconds.

One. Two. Three.

A cell phone light. That's right, I remember now. Someone was shining a cell phone light into the man's mouth, trying to light the way.

Fifty. Fifty-one.

I'm in, he said, standing, sweat on his brow.

Smiles lit the room.

He wasn't. Two minutes later, the man's heart turned fast, then flat, and he died, breathless, a dime-sized tube down his esophagus.

B is for breathing.

That's lucky. This is falling right into order.

I'm sleeping downstairs, by the furnace. It clangs and huffs. It's dry here, and the cot sags over the basement's cold concrete floor. Still, my sleeps are deep, like in my childhood, and then as now, I wake early to the smell of burning bacon and bright edges of a fading dream.

Beside me is a shelf full of *Reader's Digest*s and fishing magazines. Above these is a row of preserves, pickles, peaches, plums, in cloudy jars, echoes of my grandmother. At the foot of my bed is a workbench with a vise, a machine to put precise numbers of gunpowder grains into brass bullet casings.

A pair of antelope antlers. A photograph of my grandfather, cigarette between his fingers, the furs of fifty coyotes he caught and skinned in a single season, some hung from their noses, others stacked, empty dogs. He told me that in those dark months, he would be up before dawn, setting snares, checking them, then skin by lamplight late until he could no longer keep his eyes open. No TV. No radio. No visitors.

I climbed the creaking stairs this morning, my hand guiding my head from the low ceiling. He was at the table, mopping eggs from his plate. He's been eating that breakfast since he can remember: fried eggs, bacon, cup of thin coffee. Same on the trapline as it is here, by the lake.

He moved here when he learned that farming animals was easier than trudging beside a sled of huffing huskies collecting them. He married my grandmother, had my dad, then my uncle. From the lake at the bottom of this hill, he trawled nets filled with silver fish, fed them to snapping mink. His fur won prizes in Montreal. My dad remembers an experiment he did as a child with one of the animals who, captive her whole life, like her mother, her mother before, had never seen a living fish. He caught a perch, put it in a large tub filled with water, and released her. The mink stood on the edge, watched the perch for a moment, then bit it behind the head, killing it instantly. Forever wild.

No one needs the warmth mink coats afford anymore, not even in Canada. Fur trim on parka hoods is in style for now, at least in Toronto, but few of my friends will wear it. Some of them, I explain, won't even eat anything from an animal. Not even honey? No. My grandfather shakes his head. Such a different world.

I swirl the brown dregs of coffee in the carafe, rinse it down the sink. Past the mosaic of frost on the corners of the kitchen window, night lifts. Out of it, dark blue drifts, my car covered in snow. My grandfather coughs, and his chest rattles. In the reflection, I see him sneak a pinch of tobacco into his lip.

I remove the coffee filter and dump the grinds into the pail on the counter, already full with shells and bones. He's always known it makes less garbage to deal with if you let vegetables turn back to earth, give the fox the bones. I put on one of his coats, thick and warm, walk the pail to the food pile and a bag of trash to the burning barrel.

Behind me, flames lick papers in the burning bin and the harsh chemical smell of newsprint afire suffuses me. My breaths turn to ice. I kick the edge of the house, shake snow from one boot, then the other, step back inside, and sit at the table.

Breathing. It's second. I know, it seems like it should be first, but it's not. The first is the space necessary for it to happen, a conduit that allows for the circle, like the food pile to the fox.

There she is. Her den is right under the freezer house, where he used to store fish and skins. She comes out as soon as she knows I'm gone, lifting her paws high. She glances left, and right, picks a rib, clicks it to the angle of her jaw, and retraces her steps. Flakes soften her trail.

A breath is not an idea, like the airway, something you don't know is there until it's gone. It's the real thing, all action. Even during that flat pause between inhalation and exhalation, each cell is breathing. Your brain, your heart, each pore.

The movement is easiest to see in a heaving chest, though. With each gasp, brand-new air is pulled down our airway, towards the hot blood rushing past a thousand square feet of a sheet two cells thick, folded into our chest. Each fragile pink bubble is held open by a slick pull of negative pressure, even as we breathe out. This is why you shoot a running moose here, in the broad part of its body, just behind the foreleg.

Pow.

Its lungs, the thousands of blind bubbles no longer sucked tight to the ribs, collapse, and its front legs with it.

Breathless.

The activity of breathing never stops, but it's so natural, it shouldn't feel like work. If it does, something is wrong. Leaning on our knees, after a race, heart pounding in your ears, each breath, even if it hurts, should carry relief with the pain. If easier breaths are coming no nearer, or worse, are edging away, a person is moving in the direction of that lidless look of a narrow airway, and just past it, the drowse of last breaths.

What has been thoughtless becomes full of effort. Watch a breathless person pull up on her chest with the muscles in her neck, her jaw even. Her mouth opens like a fish's, then purses shut, trying to puff every single balloon as wide as it'll go, whatever it takes to get in a quarter-inch more air against the apartment-sized membrane in their chest.

When an infant breathes hard, a hollow dent flickers in the notch of his neck, above the first rib. If he's sick, the neck dimples sixty times a minute, maybe even higher, eighty, twice what it should be. You won't see the same worry as in an adult, though. He is too new to know how easy it should be. When he gets tired, he'll just give right up.

Once with MSF, I cared for a line of kids deciding if breathing was worth the work. I moved from bed to bed, down growing rows that stretched towards the war that is eating up breaths in Somalia, Sudan, Congo, Chad, Central African Republic, Burundi, Yemen, Syria, Mali. The children would arrive after many miles, exhausted, brothers and sisters buried in sand along the way.

At the end of each month when I was there in 2011, January, February, March, April, May, I sat in a dry office, waiting for the computer that the other sweating doctors and nurses used to tally what sick people they had seen in the weeks prior, what number of them died. Some counted pregnant women, others adults with TB. I counted people younger than twelve. Most got better. Kids are tough that way, still many days, especially as the camp grew quickly, the nurse and I would arrive after breakfast to find a small body cocooned in bright blankets.

It was difficult to know what the cause of death was, even if we were both there for it. There were no x-rays nor cultures nor blood tests. *Respiratory infection*, I would write with a shrug, flip to the next chart. If you look at world statistics, it seems that poor children die often of pneumonia, but I think some of it is just how they let go.

When oxygen is in short supply (bloop-bloooop-bloooooooop), because our lungs have collapsed or filled with water or puke or soup, or we need more air than we can grab, we make too much carbon dioxide, and our alkaline blood tips to acid. If we can't breathe it off, the tightly wound circles that work in us, unspool.

There's a look to the unravelling. My friend Bryan calls the ability to notice, in an instant, the sickest person in a crowd "the knack." It's an energetic read of a body coming apart. You can't put it into words. You see it in a person's eyes, or the way their body is held. First, there is fear, a deep knowing that the balance has been broken hard, that what has been held in so tightly, is leaking fast. Then dwindling.

Although the knack comes naturally to some, it can also be learned. It's a slow progression, starting with pieces so small they must be drawn in textbooks, then thin slices of sick cells stained red on microscope slides, to floating hearts clotted with heart attacks, pickled in formaldehyde, valves held open with pins to show webs of ruptured tendons, then whole bodies, splayed under white lights. How things come together, then how they trend apart.

Closer to the living, thought by thought, month by month, then one day, nearest yet, we start to sleep in hospitals and are assigned the newly dead. It is a rare instance where we can make a person no worse.

I was lying wide awake, like every other medical student, waiting.

Beep.

I scrambled towards the phone and perhaps, finally, the essential purpose for which I was born.

The patient in bed A-4 seems to have died. Would I come up and declare that true?

Sure, I said, shaking off my disappointment. It was a formality, I knew that, but it was still important, right? I wrapped my stethoscope around my neck, its weight still new, and walked up four flights to the internal medicine ward, room A, fourth bed.

Someone had already pulled a sheet over the person's head. A man in the facing stretcher, pretending not to look, stared at a tiny TV swivelled in front of his face, foam headphones blaring.

"Sir?" I asked, shaking the dead man's shoulder.

It felt stiff and heavy. I pulled the sheet back. A pale mouth in a final, narrow O.

"Sir?" Shake.

I felt for a pulse in his wrist. It was already cooler than it should be, drew my heat. No pulse.

I knelt, put my eyes across his chest, looking for even the smallest rise. It was still. I put a stethoscope on it. Silence.

"He's dead," I said, returning to the nurse sitting alone at the desk. He stifled a yawn, nodded.

"Dr. . . . ?" he said, flattering me, knowing that if I was really a doctor, I would be working with the living.

I walked away, down silent stairs, rubbing my fingers together, warming them, trying to loosen a memory of cooling wax that has yet to fade.

What I couldn't hear then is what I listen for now through my stethoscope's tight bell: the rush of living. Air billowing into pockets, popopopopopop, then rolling smoothly out. If normal, it sounds clear, smooth, and strong. The rhythm is regular and slow. If disturbed, you can hear the trouble, harsh and bubbling. A million Velcro gasps, of blind balloons choked by pus, or narrowed by soot.

If given the chance, oxygen floats to where it's needed. If we can't get it in, because we choke or the air is bad and filled with smoke, we become drowsy and confused, the opposite of the bubbling exhilaration we feel at the shallow end of the pool, hyperventilating before trying to swim its full length underwater.

If a person's own breath isn't enough, we can give them ours, push it past their lips using our own lungs, but you can't keep it up, no matter how long a mother would try if you asked. Better to use a bag, or a machine like a mechanical ventilator, puff out a chest, one . . . two . . . three—hold. Then out—four . . . five . . . six. It works best in the unconscious, the paralyzed, the nearly dead. No fighting the machine with breaths of their own, no biting the tube.

There are only four ventilators in Addis's largest public hospital, Black Lion. That's four more than we had in Dadaab, but it's not enough for millions of people. The machines are always in use, so in the ER we're often left splicing oxygen from a single tank, sharing it between three other patients, maybe in a badly breathing person, attaching it to a bag that we give to a family to squeeze ten times per minute. It rarely suffices. They must do nothing else, and people whose breathing takes hours to get bad need as many to get it better. Maybe more. We mostly do it when we can't bear to watch another person die right then. We do it to practise for better days.

C is for circulation.

The days are short here, this far north. The sun doesn't rise in the sky but stays within falling distance of the horizon the whole day, skims it by afternoon.

Hunting season will soon close. The ground is frozen and white, the deer scattered in bare woods, sleeping late, moving quietly. Yesterday, I sat in a tree at dawn, on our trapline, and waited for one to step into a flat clearing where I'd seen many tracks the day before. Frost sparked in midair while I looked over the barrel of my cold gun, but no deer appeared. I stayed, dutiful, until I heard the rumble of his truck, climbed down and whisked towards it through the fine snow.

"Nothing," I said, and slammed the truck door.

There isn't much time left for hunting. I leave in a few

days. I've shifts to work in Toronto, then I'm off to Addis Ababa, to help with their surplus of emergencies. Last night my grandfather advised me not to go. His argument wasn't that Ethiopia was unsafe; it was too far. Why go past the trapline? There's enough to explore there, and it's different all the time. Take last fall, the beavers dammed that creek, you know the one. The new pond goes right across the road! In those hills, there's more adventure than you'll ever get to. You don't have to search the world for it.

He is having difficulty standing from the pain in his feet. When I walked into the room this morning, he tried to push himself up from the couch. Sit, I told him, but he wouldn't, and pressed off the armrest, once, twice, winced as he stood, wobbling.

"You must want some lunch," he said, and limped, bent, into the kitchen. He calls most meals lunch, and despite having finished our second a few hours ago, he is rustling in the fridge, fixing a third.

"At least a piece of sausage," he says from around the corner.

In his mind, that I can't skin a fisher has me firmly gathered in the category of people to be helped, rather than the helpful. Even so, I persuaded him to let me see his legs this morning. He slowly removed his wool socks, put his heel, rough with callus, in my hands. I can't remember the last time I touched his bare skin.

I put my hand on the top of his foot. It was warm. I pressed his biggest toe. It blanched, then returned to pink a second later, as it should. On the top of his foot, a pulse slowly bounded.

How does it feel, I wanted to ask. Not your feet, but not walking, after so many miles?

I put his leg down.

"So," he said, pulling his socks on.

I shrugged. "Circulation seems to be OK," I said.

He nodded, his suspicion confirmed, about me, and medicine in general.

I thought it might be his vessels that were blocked. Muscles breathe, and when they're starved for oxygen, they hurt, the pain painting an arrow in the direction of a problem, like a heart attack would.

Doesn't appear that way, though, at least not from the blush of blood that flows to his toes. Could be his joints are jagged, the once smooth cartilage scarred with dots of calcium and feathered tears from falling over icy alder snags.

"You taking these?" I said, fingering a bottle of pain-killers.

"Bah," he said, waving his hand. "They don't help. I've told you, Jim, it's the bacon that keeps me alive."

When I was a boy, I watched him push a fish hook through his thumb, after I had lodged it there on a hurried cast. He did it with a pair of red needle-nose pliers, then cut the barb so he could pull the metal back through. He did it grimly, without anger, changed my hook for a new one. If he could walk through this pain, he would.

He sets a plate beside me, a piece of Ukrainian sausage on it, kielbasa, and a fresh bun, then grimaces as he lowers himself back onto the couch, puts his glasses on, and picks up a fishing magazine.

Circles. The blood moving in him now, never still, red cells tumbling over white ones, platelets too, tawny fluid with looping hormones, protein bands for making clots, dissolved air and fat and sugar, feeding his tense muscles and the joints between, the firing wires of his nerves, his wet-tasting tongue. The vessels tangle tightest at places where the most valuable work is done: the gut, the liver and lungs, back of the eye, tips of fingers.

Once air enters, our heart pushes it around with loops of feedback between our smallest parts about how the breathing project is going. With practice, you can feel two crests to the moving wave. The first, the heart pulling itself together tightly like a ball of elastics, gushing blood. The second, the living circle of arteries absorbing the push, and squeezing back.

A finger on a wrist, another on a neck, and you note a slight delay as the pulse of blood moves under an armpit, through an elbow, arrives at the hand a millisecond later than the one in the neck is flooding the brain.

For these circles, the ones that spring from them, a body needs two things to survive another five minutes: the vigorously pounding piston of our heart, and pressure enough to pass fluid through the mess of fine, hot wires and have it come back.

When you shoot an animal as large as a moose, you should cut its neck right there, spill as much blood as you can into the ground. Otherwise, the muscles get stiff and chewy with clot. A few winters ago, while my brother walked a mile away, I startled a moose in the thick bush. We were both surprised. The animal jerked his heavy head from the tip of a small tree, turned, and ran. I aimed at that spot behind its foreleg, and fired.

I couldn't tell if I'd hit him, so I charged hard on his

trail. Branches stung my face. At the bottom of a short hill, his legs buckled. I slowed, and skidded down the frosty leaves to where he lay. His nostrils flared air in great white huffs. Blood drained down the brown fur of his neck. I shot him in the head and his great bowl of horns tipped to the side. I drew my knife, but hesitated. My brother crashed through the brush, saw me standing there, took out his knife, bent forward, and cut the big vessels in the animal's throat.

"Go get Dad."

We crawled into his chest and scooped insides out until it was hollow, sawed his head off, then broke him into pieces small enough to carry from the bush. We hung the legs, the ribs, and back in the old freezer building across from this window, far out of reach of the weasels and mice that, whiskers twitching, sniffed blood in the air.

It took about five days for red to stop pattering onto the newspapered floor, and only then did the butchering begin. In the days leading up to that big work, we ate the liver, the kidneys, the tongue, the once living heart.

If a vessel opens, from a cut, or bullet, and is not closed, the heart runs dry. If it's a nick or a scrape, a mesh of proteins and platelets can do the work, leap into the breach, staunch it, form a thin skin until a thicker one grows over it in a few days. If the hole's too big, the blood's web can't hold the pressure back.

Once, a welder arrived to me pale and dead because the man he worked beside watched a metal sheet fall and slice his partner's upper arm, and instead of applying pressure, to keep the blood inside, he left the room to call an ambulance.

He should have taken off his shirt and pressed firmly, like a platelet would, onto the hole, then, if the blood continued to drain, leaned on the wound with more of his weight and if that wasn't working, fuck it, tie a belt above it, just tight enough for the bleeding to stop. The body beyond would have starved from a lack of air, would even die if without it too long, and the guy may have lost his welding arm after all, but at least he could have been sitting up in bed, staring at his stump, instead of lying on the trauma stretcher dead white and much too cold.

If the cut is on the head, neck, or torso, pressure is all you can do, until a surgeon with microscope loupes over her eyes brings things back together.

Meanwhile the circle the heart pushes into, if alive, knows just what to do. It opens in places that need more flow, closes off in ones that don't. In that man, dying alone with his friend on the phone, the heart beat faster and faster while the circle of vessels started to slowly shrink, and his fingers, then hands, feet then legs, turned mottled while the last drab of blood shot to his brain, kidneys, liver, finally, his heart.

Thud-d. Thud-d. Thud-d.

That's a heart's sound. Not from its knock on the ribs, but from its valves snapping shut snapping shut snapping shut so blood won't fall back through and ruin all its work

If the heart beats wrong, too fast or too slow, stops, vessels relax, fatten and coil, blood cools and thickens, capillaries start to leak, cells starve then die. There's no breath to move, no bigger story to tell.

One afternoon, about ten years ago, a neighbour found my grandfather slumped over the steering wheel of his pickup, at the top of the hill, his arm out the window. His heart had slowed almost to a stop. When he was pulled from his seat and laid on the ground, blood washed to his brain, and he regained consciousness. He tried to sit up, and fainted.

The neighbour and a friend carried him to the same couch he's on now, and from it, he waved away everyone who suggested the hospital, until my grandmother arrived. He went. They hooked him up to the electrocardiogram, saw that the fast flicker in the atrium, its route scarred by tobacco smoke or some ancestral gene, wasn't carrying to the ventricles, which, without encouragement, assume a pace too lazy to make much pressure. He went by ambulance to the nearest city and got a pacemaker an hour after he arrived.

Like a great magic, electricity arrives spontaneously in the heart and holds us together. Once it leaves a body, though, there's no bringing it back. If there's a little left, even if confused, there is a chance. If you get there in time, a few minutes, say, and find a buzz in the heart, the cells can be reminded about the direction of their work if you run a current quickly through them, causing a single violent contraction.

This is the scene in a medical drama when someone shouts, "Is everybody clear?" before a patient's body jerks. The shock is like lightning, gone in an instant, and only aligns what electricity is already there. It can only help people with a charge of their own, who have blood to push and a heart strong enough to do it. If there is no flicker, we see only a flat line. The EKG leads might as well be attached to the wall.

Although in the ER there are supplements for a body's "A," a breathing tube for instance, and for "B," lips or bags or ventilators, there is nothing near as good as a heart. If someone drops, pulseless, newly dead, you can push from the outside, with CPR, use your energy to buy time until you find electricity. At its most vigorous, CPR provides one-quarter of the flow a person needs to live. The patient's brain is dying, kidneys and liver too, just more slowly.

Every minute without a full pulse, a future leaks away. If a heart stops in hospital, with people around to leap on the chest right away, one in four walk back into their lives. On the streets of cities with people trained to do it, and ambulances to call, one in ten.

In the ER, we never know which one we might have in front of us, so if there's a small chance to rescue a future, we intervene. We shock, we pace the heart, give blood, break ribs, use drugs to move what's left of our five litres to the centre for one more push to the brain in case what kindles the electricity catches.

The drugs we use are similar to the adrenalin that surges when you're walking down a dark alley and two men step from the shadows, same as what wakes me up, panting, deep from a dream where I'm pounding wildly on ice to free my frozen brother. The heart speeds, the pressure hammers, pupils widen to allow in as much light as possible, because death is near and we must see more clearly than ever before whether to fightfightfight or runrunrun. For some of us, our last sensation will be of being fully, forcefully alive.

D is for drugs.

I went into his bedroom today, to fetch pills, and found it filled with my grandmother's things. A string of pearls dangled from a mirror. There were notes to herself in a tight librarian's script stacked on the desk, and a closet filled with her clothes. It was like walking into a memory, everything familiar, but a fragment of the living thing.

She's been gone a year now. My whole life, she was the person I most wanted to see. I told her things I have never told anyone, my dreams and secrets. She persuaded the druggist in town to not burn unsold comics after he had torn their covers off to send back for a refund. I had boxes and boxes of the most coveted editions, none worth a penny. It's how I learned to read.

Her last months, she spent in hospital, my grandfather

beside her, watching her fall away. First her will, then her memories, her senses, then her breath. My mom says nurses still talk about how he sat there, every moment, right to the end.

I wasn't there for it. Too far, I would tell myself, and then board a plane for the other side of the world.

The last time I saw her, she was still at home, writing her notes, walking up and down these steep stairs that are difficult for me to climb. She got a nosebleed that wouldn't quit with pressure, so I took her to the small hospital where, one day, she would die. The doctor recommended liquid cocaine to stop the blood. The drug squeezes vessels shut and at the same time numbs the skin, so if you burn a weeping spot, a person won't even wince.

The nurse put the soaked cotton ball into my grandmother's nostril. She closed her eyes and leaned back. Her face was white, shiny under the lights. A river of blood leaked to the corner of her mouth. I dabbed it away with a tissue.

A minute or so later, her lids fluttered open, and a brightness returned. "I feel much better," she said. "Let's go home."

There is no drug that has an effect that doesn't have a side effect. As cocaine numbs the nose, it makes things seem better than they are.

"Not quite yet," I answered. "But soon."

The doctor came into the room, fished a cautery stick from a black pouch.

I took the bottle of pills from beside my grandfather's bed.

I'm trying harder than ever to be helpful. He doesn't like to drive far, especially on icy roads, so yesterday I drove him to his old farm, around where he and my grandmother first met, a hundred kilometres from here. His world is slowly shrinking with his body, but his mind still roams.

This morning, my final act: doctoring. It's something I do only rarely for those I'm close to. Although love is the best ground to act from, it helps to have distance during difficult decisions. From errors too.

I hand my grandfather his pills. He uncorks the plastic bottle, spills out the tablets on the table, breaks one, puts a half in his mouth, drops the other half back. I open the drawer where he keeps the rest of the drugs. A dozen round bottles roll in tight circles.

"How do you know which ones to take?"

"I remember."

I gather them, study their labels. "These are bad. Also bad," I say, lining them up on the counter. "These ones are OK," I say, and pick two of the cloudy orange containers. "They're for pain. Oval one in the morning, when you wake up. Two of these white ones around lunch."

I shake out an oval one. He nods, puts it between his lips, swallows it with water. I scratch instructions on the bottles, draw a calendar on a blank piece of paper, with names and shapes.

All these loose pills clattering around, tiny writing on the labels. They should be bundled together by the pharmacy, a week's worth, into a blister pack, timed right, easy to take.

As we get older, more conditions appear for which medicines have been made, but there are fewer years to capture their effects, so mistakes matter more, side effects rise and combine. Do no harm is our most important rule, but we break it all the time trying to do good.

A teacher in medical school insisted that anyone I admitted to hospital should have all their drugs stopped, so we could reintroduce the fewest a person needed, one at a time. Good medicine, she said, was getting out of the body's way as much as possible. From her I learned the most productive question I ask in the ER when someone tells me they feel sick: what have we done to you?

"Why do you have so many?" I ask my grandfather.

He shrugs. "It's what they give me."

Heart specialist. Kidney specialist. Bone doctor. They add a drug or two that they know well, and the person and their family doctor are stuck watching the list grow, reluctant to winnow any, in case there is a benefit neither of them see.

I saw a man once, on twenty-two different medicines. They were bundled into foil pods like a space-age meal, to be eaten throughout the day. He was lying in bed, waxen. He could barely move. That's a lot of pills, man, I said. He shrugged. Is it?

I line the bottles up. Looking at when they were prescribed, how many are left, I can tell which ones he takes, what he has given up on. I pluck from them what he really needs.

These three. One to prevent gout, one for blood pressure, and a baby aspirin.

Needs might be too strong a word. More help than hurt. Aspirin, so reliable that we have paramedics give it in the backs of ambulances if there is a hint of a heart attack, and over the millennia that doctors have been telling patients to eat it, despite billions of dollars of trying, we've not developed one better. Even so, if one hundred people like my grandfather took it every day for two years, it might save two of them a heart attack. Which two bodies, we don't know, we haven't yet the math, so we play averages, err on the cautious side, and the other ninety-eight get the cost and some bleeding noses.

The blood pressure medicine helps half as many, about one in a hundred, but makes nine so sick they must stop taking it. By the time you're here, at "D," the threads you pull to keep things moving can be so thin they start to disappear. Quantity of life, smoothed out over millions, is easier to show than what makes one worth living.

For the gout, well, taking the pill does little better than nothing at all, but I know he hates that pain so much, he won't want to quit it.

I pull a bottle of antinauseants from the lineup, draw a big X on the lid, another on the label. These are sedating. When crossing the floor becomes your greatest peril, you must be alive to small edges.

"Take these to your doctor. Tell him: no more."

"I don't eat those ones. They make me feel bad."

Eighty years ago, near here, a train tipped off the tracks while it was rolling full speed. Its cars skidded and buckled, and the cargo flipped into the bush. My grandfather and his brother, long dead now, found a case from the wreck. In it were unbroken bottles of whisky. They finished one between them, staggered home, and fell into bed, dead drunk. It was their first time. At dawn, they were roused for their daily chores. They spent the day vomiting. My grandfather hasn't been drunk since. He's not against it, necessarily, just doesn't know why a guy would bother to do it. How could something that made you worse get you better?

I bind all the pill bottles that weren't helping with a fat elastic band. "You don't need these ones."

"Good."

I put them back in the drawer, grab my keys from the table, put them on the kitchen counter. I'm leaving in a few hours. Slowly my things are shifting to the door, then the porch with its chill of winter air. I stand to do the dishes.

"Sit, sit. I'll take care of them. I need something to do."

I listen.

"Game of crib?" I ask.

"You ready to lose?"

"There's always a first time."

My hand is terrible. It's tough to decide between the worst cards, but I choose two, throw them on the table, face down. He wins most of the games, unless I get particularly lucky with the draw. His style of play is unpredictable. He will forsake points almost randomly, making probability impossible to anticipate. He leads with a ten. I don't know what he's thinking. I match it.

"Twenty for two."

He plays another ten.

"Thirty for six."

His brass pegs inch ahead of my silver ones. His hands, thick and lined, sweep away the fallen cards.

Maybe just a small amount of sedative.

One of the pain medicines I chose is metabolized by the kidney. He has just one. It's something I might avoid in a person I knew less well. I gave a small dose, enough in the morning so he can stand at the stove, and maybe in the early afternoon, imagine the stairs, his workbench below. I know him and what makes his life worth living. Bacon. Tomorrow-bacon, not maybe-bacon three years from now.

Cards patter. He scoops his, decides in a glance.

When I was learning how to practise where there were few doctors and no hospitals, setting up clinics under a tree, a mentor reminded me to give everyone at least some pills, even if only vitamins. If I didn't, he said, they would think I was holding back, and go elsewhere when their children were really sick. At the end of a day, I watched them walk down the dusty road, trading tablets back and forth, a red for a yellow.

It is a rare person who waits two hours in the ER, or under a tree, when told that no medicine invented will heal her better than her own body, considers the answer the marvel it is, so most of us give out medicines pulled from a category of vague drugs that don't work that well but don't hurt much either. Antacids. Something for nausea. Cough suppressants. Antidepressants. Many of them just make a person sleepy, and everyone feels better after a nap, or they occupy the mind, let it rest from some of its worry, because with rest and time, in well-fed, healthy people, healing usually happens.

Selling drugs to people with money is the fastest way to make money that mankind has found. We spend more money on them than anything but food and shelter. In the West, we swallow them by the ton, whether they do us any good or not, and they move through our bodies into our water supply, for everyone to drink. In the Potomac River, there is enough estrogen from birth control pills that fish switch sexes. Salmon caught off the east coast are made of, at least partly, cocaine, antidepressants, and blood thinners.

The garbage can in the office I share with a dozen other ER doctors is filled with unopened mail from drug companies. They try every way to flash a new name in front of my eyes on official-looking paper, so it flutters about in our subconscious, finds its way onto a prescription pad without my really thinking about it. They sponsor conferences, and give us pens, pay us if we let them. They play, in the end, to a weakness. If it can be proved, at great expense, that an existing medicine can be improved, so that it is easier to take or remember, does less harm or more good for a few more people in a hundred thousand, even at twice the cost, we lean towards it, and with us, millions of patients and their dollars with little consideration of how the money might be better spent.

We are told, increasingly, that healthcare must run like a business, the patients like customers, that they must leave pleased. People feel better with a prescription in their hand, and if there's even a small chance a pill might help, why not try? Relief gleams brighter than a possible hurt, and by the time a bad outcome emerges, so much has happened, it is tough to know what to blame, sickness or cure.

A drug's means to facilitate lasting change is often disappearingly small because a body is in constant flux with its environment, external and internal, emotional, social, and genetic, each so intimately connected that you couldn't draw a line where one starts and the other ends.

Altering a single physiological process affects only a facet easiest to measure, a test parameter, a blood glucose or pressure, the serotonin level in a brain. The ability of this adjustment to influence a person's life is often weaker than we let on. Nor can we anticipate the spiralling effects that loop from it.

Despite all the white coats peering into microscopes, we don't know straightforward things, like the fewest days a person with pneumonia should poison their body with antibiotics so the bacteria pulling it apart find something else to eat.

Already, on our skin, in our stomachs, there are more bacteria than cells in our bodies, and these animals eat the drug too. Some die—helpful ones, others just along for the ride. In their wake, some of the ones that cause disease stick around, resistant, mix with the ones that helped us stay well, waiting for another chance to grow. On hospital doorknobs, some bacteria cling, resistant to every drug man has made because we've used them too long, in cattle feed and in people who never needed them.

Some medicines save lives. Thyroid hormone in people who have none, insulin in a dependent diabetic, HIV antivirals, some chemotherapies, antimalarials, antibiotics in serious bacterial infections, steroids to quell an immune system on fire. Powerful ones are lined up right now, row on row, in a brightly lit room in my Toronto ER. Should we need one that is missing, a pharmacist flies it to us through a pneumatic tube.

They are so strong, conversation in the space where they are mixed is discouraged so nurses don't transpose names like adenosine and atropine. The first, if your heart is racing when it shouldn't, will stop it so flat, just like that, only for a few seconds, but long enough that people fear they're dying. The second makes people feel their heart is leaping out of their chest, and if you came in with a heart too slow to make a pulse, we'd put that atropine in you in seconds, maybe even right through your jeans. It's not as fast as the glands on your kidneys can spill adrenalin, but we practise, and each year, we get a bit faster.

In Addis, I'll see a teenager with a heart so sick, he is on medicines for old men, drugs that to any doctor read like an elegy. Warfarin, digoxin, spironolactone, ashes to ashes. He had rheumatic fever when he was young, easily prevented by treating strep throat with penicillin. Although, like pneumonia, we might not know the minimum number of days he needed it for, he needed at least some. This is math we have. While we are making drugs that don't help much, but don't hurt much either, people who need some of what we dump down the drain, die.

We have Adrenalin in Ethiopia, a few rolling vials in a particular drawer. Some Valium, for those who are seizing, or can't calm down, magnesium for pregnant women with sky-high blood pressure. No adenosine, though, not yet. Working on that. I've stopped short of bringing vials from Canada, though it's hard to teach without it.

"You're in trouble now," he says, his pegs a few holes away from the end.

"Part of my strategy."

Another bad hand.

Hundreds of drugs are in development for adult-onset diabetes, one not much better than the other, none more useful than eating differently and walking for half an hour a day but so profitable that our brightest minds are pulled towards the dollars. It's too bad, because there is an effect beyond the drug, and it requires a person's belief that help is on offer. When an intention to heal is met with the will of a person to get well: catalysis. If neither is there, no pills can conjure it, at least not for long.

I'll see one day. That type of diabetes is in my family. Maybe it will run right through to me. Wonder if I'll take the drug. Maybe. I guess I'll see how it makes me feel.

"One more?"

"I should probably get moving."

"All right."

I put the pills back in the drawer, sweep crumbs from the table with one hand into the other, then throw them in the pail.

I'm packed. I didn't bring much. My things are by the door. The lake is frozen. Soon it will be covered, and snow will drift and blow for months. It's going to be a long winter. It will be difficult for him to move.

"I'll be OK," he says. We have a rough hug at the door, and I climb into my parents' car, to head south in their direction.

I wait for the car to warm, and see him pass by the small window my grandma used to peer out, smiling, waving. My grandfather doesn't linger, and his image is gone in a second.

E is for emergency.

The sleep before my night shift is fitful. The thump of bass from the marijuana café that shares my bedroom wall works its way onto that wire that plays between my heart and mind, tightens it, and I turn in tangled sheets. So many years of night shifts, still that excited fear.

My alarm blinks on, showers my room with blue light. I use two now, after Dave slept through his, was woken up by police officers at his door, sent to make sure he was still alive. I roll from bed, pull on my clothes, set water to boil for coffee.

A sleep headache dully throbs behind my eyes as I ride my bike downtown through back alleys and side streets. Snow melts brown across streetcar tracks waiting to catch my tire. A last turn, and ambulance lights flash.

I weave through the queue. Slush spatters to my knees, as I lock my bike to a yellow fence. On the sidewalk stained with fading blots of blood, a man smokes. I pass him without a word, and the doors swing open, blow hot air past me into the winter.

Yellow backboards for cradling broken spines litter the hall. Another swinging door, and the noise of the waiting room crashes.

". . . . . . blood pressure. . . . . . Wong, Margaret Wong to registration. . . . . health card. . . . . (hisss). . . . . beepbeepbeep. . . ."

Two medics, a person belted on a folding stretcher between them, heart monitor alarming, wait for the attention of a registration clerk paper-clipping patient charts behind glass an inch thick.

A man in a jean jacket sits in one of the two triage chairs, waving sheets of paper. Jen, a nurse, sits across from him, on the other side of a half-door, no glass for her. She needs to touch people, feel their pulse, smell their breath. She nods, *yes*, *yes*, catches my eye and waves.

I smile. She is in the middle of a decision that will determine, based on his story—how he appears, how quickly his pulse bounds—which part of the ER he will be sent to, major, intermediate, or minor, and what his place in line will be there. Anyone with that many medical papers in his hand is used to lines. I'll be seeing him in minor.

"Hey, Doc," the security guard says, thumbs hooked in his flak vest, standing a few paces away, watching the man wave his papers, making sure he stays calm. At least three guards are assigned to our ER, more minutes away.

So many drugs downtown makes for unpredictable people. One of my colleagues was taken hostage once, and the assailant, waving a gun, was shot in the waiting room by a SWAT team. As soon as he fell, he was rushed to the trauma room. They couldn't save him. SWAT teams rarely miss. Since that day, our security is serious.

"Buzz me in?" I ask. He reaches behind his shielded desk.

I pass the waiting room. It's full. Police sit on either side of a prisoner in an orange jumpsuit, head in his hands, ankle chains dropping in a grey puddle between his feet. A woman pinches her nose, her head tilted back. Another set of medics lean on a stretcher, chatting to the old woman buckled into it. People in chairs glance up, in case I'm someone who might call their name. When they see it's not a nurse, they turn back to their phones.

I walk down the minor hall. A man with an IV draining into his wrist, and a red, swollen leg. More people in chairs.

The minor desk has their charts piled to its end. Carolyn, a nurse, adds another, sees me, smiles in sympathy. I shrug. A drunk man shouts from a stretcher behind her and struggles to sit up.

"Settle down!" she says. "I told you I'd be with you in a minute."

He quiets. Tough love here, but it's true.

I pass out of the ER, towards the change room. It is quiet again. It is one of the pleasures of night shifts. So few people work them, you find solidarity with the ones who do, awake and purposeful in a dark, dreaming city.

The scrubs machine whirrs, then clanks. I pull a pair from its white, shifting rows, take off my street clothes, replace them with anonymous green. I put on my ID, a stethoscope around my neck, its weight familiar now, steal a black pen from Fernando's desk next to mine.

Down the empty back hallway, full during the day with people puzzling at signs on the wall, a man spins wax onto an already shining floor.

Emergency Department. Authorized personnel only.

I place my badge on the automatic door.

Click.

Major. Bright lights glare harshly from every corner. At the consultants' desks, teams of residents pore over lab tests, scroll over screens looking for a pattern that would fit into a diagnosis. One takes off his glasses and puts his head on the desk. Beside him, a colleague, blinking sleepily, stares at an x-ray of a chest, white bones frozen on a computer screen.

That once was me, but since I graduated my residency, no one's looking over my shoulder to catch mistakes, and I no longer work such long hours, but I do work a range of shifts. Christmas afternoon, midnight on a Sunday, if not me, someone like me. In eight-hour intervals, we cover the clock. From dawn until midnight there are four or five of us scattered through the ER, another waiting by the phone for a serious trauma, but nights, no matter how special they seem at the start, no one wants to work them. Eventually, research says, they make you sick, something you didn't need science to tell you, so in the smallest hours, you work alone.

And quickly. As cities pile people downtown, as people live longer on more medicines that make more side effects, have more surgeries and more complications, as specialization break bodies into smaller and smaller parts, as our population spends more time on screens than outside and grows ever more anxious, there are more people in our ER every day.

Worried people tap a symptom into search engines instead of asking their grandmother, and like it was when I was in medical school, before I learned that diseases make particular patterns in a sick body not a well one, they assign themselves the worst possible disease.

When I was a student, I felt a single lymph node on the back of my neck, the size of a pea. It's still there. My heart leapt when I read about lymphoma. I most surely had it. My vision blurred during neuroanatomy lab, and while the class was colouring nerve tracts, I approached the neurosurgeon at the front, told him gravely about my tumour. He told me to sit back down. A migraine headache. My vision cleared. Sicknesses make you feel sick. That's why young children are such a pleasure to treat. Their mind has yet to learn to deny their bodies.

Only a few years ago, it was rare to see two hundred people register. Now, we rarely have fewer. Soon, we'll need two of us at night. As it is now, we run all night and never get caught up

Tom sits at the major desk, looking at a virtual map of the department on a computer screen. Each room is red, meaning full. I put my coffee mug beside him.

"How's it goin'?" I ask, snatch a piece of paper from a printer's tray.

"Living the dream," he says, stretching his arms above him, and yawns.

A young woman in a white coat hovers five paces away.

"Are you the medical student on tonight?"

She nods.

"Well, gather close" I say, and flop into a chair.

"You have a senior resident around here too," Tom says. "She was what some people call 'on time.'"

"Fascinating. Why?"

"You'll have to ask her. She's seeing somebody already."

"That's a good sign."

"Yeah, she's great. I worked with her the other day. OK, I gotta get out of here . . ."

I pull closer.

"Bed one is a seventy-year-old man with a history of heart failure, came in about an hour ago, quite short of breath. Looked pretty bad at first, but he turned around with nitro and some diuretics. He doesn't even need oxygen anymore."

I nod. Nitroglycerin lets veins fatten, drops the load rushing into the heart such that it can beat more easily. Diuretics kick salt from our kidneys, and with it, the extra water from a failed heart that has leaked across the membrane of our lungs.

"Chest x-rays . . . here."

He pulls up a silhouette of the man's ribs, plump heart in the middle. The lungs, usually as invisible as the air they hold, are whiter where fluid has seeped from the pressures of a failing pump.

"Not bad," I say, pointing out to the medical student where Tom and I are looking.

"Turns out he hasn't been taking his pills, and we talked about that. Still waiting on blood work, but if he passes a walk test, I think he should be able to go with follow-up."

These ten minutes are the most dangerous ones in the ER. I haven't seen any of the people Tom is talking about. I will if asked, but there are new people in beds, more every few minutes. You need to trust the person who is leaving that their plans are good, that they insert no false certainty.

Tom has the knack. And the account makes sense, the details tie into each other. If they didn't, we would go over it again, or he would ask me to start anew.

"Bed two is a thirty-five-year-old man . . ."

I scratch down fifteen short stories of people's lives, into a line or two of worries, circle the ones with outstanding business.

"This your first night shift here . . . Zainab?" I ask the medical student, looking at her badge

"Yes."

"Well, that's exciting," I say, standing up and walking around the nursing desk to the charts of the patients waiting to be seen. She follows.

"OK. So, quickly. All these beds"—I gesture to the semicircle of curtains around us—"are major."

She nods.

"Sicker people. Heart attacks, or things that could be them. Strokes and overdoses. Traumas. Low blood pressures, hearts that are too fast or too slow. The unconscious. People who need constant monitoring, because they're getting sicker, or because the information gathered over time helps us know whether it's safer for them to stay in hospital or whether they can go home."

I point to a screen that collects a dozen different hearts, beating at different paces.

"Say if someone comes in from a fall, and they're not sure if they tripped or fainted. We watch to make sure their heart isn't skipping beats. You can scroll back—like this—for however long they've been hooked up. Cool, right?"

"Yes," she said.

"If they have a home, that's where we send them, if it's safe to. If it's not, or they need treatment only found in hospital, they're admitted. There are more nurses here in major, like one for every two beds. That's what makes the difference between here and intermediate. We take over those rooms at one a.m. People are on monitors there, but have fewer nurses to check on them, less time per sick person."

A woman in a white coat comes out of bed 11 and joins us. I smile in greeting.

"Just orienting Zainab to the ER. In intermediate, we see abdominal pain, kidney stones. Vaginal bleeding. That type of thing. People with mostly normal vital signs, who can wait for an hour or two, though they often wait longer. We also have a security guard there at all times, so that's where we put people who are psychotic, suicidal, or high on drugs. Drug-wise, here at St. Mike's . . . a lot of crystal these days for some reason. Some crack, but everything really. GHB, MDMA, heroin, fentanyl, OxyContin." I stop to think. "And booze. Lots of booze. People can be pretty agitated, so best to check with me or one of the nurses before you go into a room alone."

Zainab follows my eyes, hangs off my words. I was the same. It was the most exciting place I had been.

"Last, minor. It's the busiest. Only a couple nurses,

little monitoring. Long waits, small problems. Well, to us. To the person, worst day of their life."

The senior resident smiles, nods.

"Here's how it will work. You"—I point to Zainab—"will see cases, do the history and physical exam, talk to me about what you think is going on, and we'll come up with a treatment plan together. Make sense? And you"—I flip the senior resident's badge the right way round, Ellen, visiting final-year resident, on a trauma rotation, maybe wants a job—"talk to me before you order any scans or discharge anybody home. We'll connect every hour or so to see what's going on. If any traumas come in, they're all yours."

"Great."

"Oh yeah, and if either of you hear 'Dr. Maskalyk to wherever,' meet me there. Something exciting is happening."

They nod, satisfied.

"OK, break. We'll work in major for a bit, then let the other docs go home."

I shuffle through the clipboards of patients yet to be seen. Chest pain. Shortness of breath. Confused. The names become secondary. People assume their sickness and the number of their bed.

"Here you go," I say, hand Zainab the chart on top. "Chest pain. Sounds scary." She walks to bed 8, stands outside its curtain, studying the red electrocardiogram.

"I worked with her the other day in minor," Tom says, from over my shoulder, as he gathers the wide scatter of his papers. "She's solid too."

"Nice. Good sleep."

I look through the remaining charts. Confused, registered at 2323 hours. Shortness of breath, 2340. It's best to not get picky about what you see, just go to whoever's next.

A preference for the sickest, though. That's what matters most, shuffles the order. The triage nurse makes a first fast pass, glancing at the vital signs, heart rate, blood pressure, temperature, but also how the body is held, the clothes, the worry, asks a few critical questions about chest pain, how suddenly the weakness started.

The inspection continues in finer detail when the patient moves into a room and another nurse spends more minutes on the story, pulling out details, sees them gasp as they change into a gown, what bruises are revealed, then comes back in twenty minutes to note what's changed. The worst sicknesses don't stay still. Short of breath then gulping for it, the confused turn unconscious.

A person tells the story a third time to me, about how they came to be hooked to all these machines. Some get frustrated, but I need to hear it myself. I must be forever suspicious, trust no previous information necessarily, at least not more than what I can gather. I have diagnosis and treatment in mind, decide who gets discharged or referred for admission, the middle and end of their emergency department story. In the eyes of the law, my mistakes matter most, so I ask two questions in enough different ways that the answers are as clear as possible: what exactly are you here for, and why, exactly, today?

Then I look at their shoes. In truth, I probably look at them first, and if they have none, their feet. It tells me how much money they have, what kind of care I can expect them to afford their body once they leave.

Once my teachers left me alone with badly breathing bodies, once they knew I could tell a heart that should be shocked from one better slowed, how unlikely someone with bare feet, black with asphalt, would be to follow up, my work was to know the emergency department. Which bed to keep free for people who are quickly dying, which nurse to call for an IV in a drowsy infant.

Regardless of which bed they start in, the sickest win their way to the front, and we see them first, then everyone else in the order they come, as fast as we can. I say that sentence so often to people frustrated at the wait, I want it flashing underneath "Emergency." Maybe beside it, a neon palm tree, for some good vibes.

We won't change what we do for the richest, or the loudest, or the person who woke up early to get in line before we opened, but we'll move whatever way we need to accommodate the weakest. The ER has the best logic of any place I know. It's why I work here. It's something to believe in.

I drain the rest of my coffee. One of the nurses turns the lights down. Some of the patients Tom saw are numb, drowsing, morphine washing through their brains, waiting for admission orders to be written by the resident with his head on the desk. It's quiet, at least for now, but you must never, ever say that word in this ER. It is our one superstition. Well, we haven't a bed 13, so I suppose there are two.

I walk past the man in bed 1. He breathes easily. A body in bed 6 clicks and whirrs on a ventilator, paralyzed and unconscious. Space is being made for her in the intensive care unit. In the rare event there wasn't some, she would be flown to another ICU by helicopter, maybe even wake up in a brand-new city once she could gather her own breaths again. What a surprise.

Around the ER, in major, intermediate, minor, in bright rooms, twenty families sit, anxious. For them, hours of waiting. For us, a series of five-minute encounters until morning.

I stand outside the bed of the confused man. I have seen so many people pass through this bed. Seizing ones. Bleeding ones. A man yelling, bug-eyed, high on amphetamines, while security strained to hold him down.

I glance at his chart. Eighty-six. I pull the curtain aside.

He looks older. He is alone, his eyes closed, mouth drawn over empty gums. His face is freshly shaven.

Who did it? I wonder. So careful. Not even a nick. I lean closer. The smell of aftershave.

Maybe he did it himself.

No stridor. Oxygen in his blood was good, at 98 per cent. His heart tracing is slow and regular on the black screen. He could wait minutes. I shuffle the next chart forward.

Bed 14. Shortness of breath. I draw its curtain back, and the face of a man I have seen half a dozen times looks up. He sits, shirtless, legs dangling, sharp shoulders rounded forward, heaving up and down. His nose flares as he draws in a breath, cheeks blow fat as he puffs it out past the edges of an oxygen mask connected from his face to the wall.

"Hey . . . Doc . . ."

"Saeed. Asthma again?"

"Yeah."

"Still smoking?"

"Cuttin' . . . down . . . five . . . a day . . ."

"Good." I put the bell of my stethoscope on his back. Wheezes. "You coughing anything up? Fevers? Using your puffers?"

No's. I scribble an order on his chart for inhaled medicines, a steroid pill to shrink the inflammation in his scarred lungs. In an hour, he will walk out of here with an inhaler in his pocket and a prescription for more. Same every time. He always says he needs more. He must have a hundred of the things. What's happened to them all? I don't ask.

I drop the orders off at the nursing station, walk back to the bed of the confused man.

"Sir!" I shout. He doesn't blink. I move to his ear. "Sir!"

Nothing. I rap his chest. No response. More "unconscious" than "confused." I rub my knuckles hard, back and forth, on his sternum. He grimaces, moves his hands to mine. Good. Something is infinitely better than nothing.

I feel for a pulse in the arm that clutches mine. The skin at his wrist is paper-thin. Skin does that as we age, fades, its fat and elastics grow loose. Sometimes older people come in after bumping their shins and the skin will just have peeled away. Putting it back together is like sewing wrapping paper; the threads just slide right through. I've learned to use tape.

Between his tendons, a pulse bounds. He snores quietly. His breath smells of denture paste.

I look more carefully at the chart. From nursing home. Alzheimer's. History of stroke. Two-person transfer. Not eating, not drinking × 3 days. Blood sugar normal. No family. End-of-life form signed by public trustee: transfer to hospital, antibiotics OK. Do not resuscitate.

The murmur of voices carries through the curtain.

I've seen this man before too. Versions of him, I mean, so many I've lost count, all of them dead now.

I saw two roads when I noted his age and complaint. Review his medicines for sedatives, order blood work, chest x-ray, test for urinary tract infection, a CAT scan of the head to look for blood that, if seen, will cause me to stop the aspirin he's on.

Or let him die. He's on his way. Whatever fear of death we're treating by pretending to stave it off, this man isn't feeling it. If I could talk to him, I don't know if he would want to stretch this part of his life. But I can't.

That's the tension that pulls through this place. Not just how to call out the right medicine over a dozen other voices and have the right person hear it, or not to miss a tiny white patch of blood on a CAT scan when you're blinking sleepily at 4 a.m., but how to mete out the great wealth to those who might profit in ways that matter. Admitting to intensive care all the people who will never again open their eyes would fill it in a day. Pour blood into people who won't stop bleeding and you'll run dry while they'll still die. These decisions become more real in places like Ethiopia, where for a single person there may be two units of blood to spare, not twenty.

I pull the oxygen nasal prongs tighter around the man's ears.

A nurse pushes the curtain aside, squinting at what I've written on Saeed's chart. "What does this say?"

"Umm . . . Ventolin, 5 milligrams." I pull the old man's sheet back to the top of his chest.

"Wow. Every year, your writing gets worse and worse."

"You gotta learn to love the mystery."

"I don't," she says, and walks away.

I pull the man's lower lids down. The pupils tighten briskly in a blue iris, clouded with cataracts from the sun's rays.

Someone's son, brother, father, husband, lover. Grandfather. One day, someone will bend to my wrinkled face, put a stethoscope on this chest, and listen to my heart pound down, their mind on their own private thoughts while mine dances with memories flown through tiny holes.

Or maybe I'll be surrounded by people I love. Or be alone on the floor.

I swish the curtain aside and leave the room.

Zainab asks questions of a patient in another bed.

Twenty minutes to one.

In Ethiopia, my friends are just waking up. They are seven hours ahead, seven years behind. Coptic calendar. Direct flight Toronto to Addis. One sleeping pill, wake up in the motherland. I can't wait to see them. Their eyes will light up. Mine too.

Emergency medicine is new there. In the country's largest public hospital, the one that caters to the poorest people, the ones with no options to visit the private clinics that pepper the streets around it, the first group of men and women are being taught to deliver the promise of sickest first. Four of them will become the country's first emergency doctors, the first teachers of medicine that matters when minutes do.

Last time I was there, Demelesh stopped me, early one morning, on my way to the ER. Dr. James, he said, eyes red with fatigue but bright. Last night, a man came in, his heart stopped, and we shocked him, and today he is alive!

He grinned from ear to ear.

I drop my orders into the box, fill out a requisition for the CAT scan.

A nurse leaves the medication room with the medicines for Saeed. Behind her, alphabetical shelves of intravenous and oral drugs. On every square inch of wall, plugs, oxygen spigots, metal carts with bottles of saline, iodine, chlorhexidine, hydrogen peroxide, sterile non-latex gloves, masks to fit any face, clean kits with long, thin needles to thread between vertebrae, machines to warm bodies, ones to cool them down, restraints for the violent, charcoal for the poisoned, everything within twenty metres of where I stand, and what isn't here is run to us in the hands of a huffing porter.

Zainab and I discuss the chest-pain case. Thirty-six-year-old man, otherwise well, sharp pain, off and on for a week, lasting a few seconds. The electrocardiogram traces a normal heart.

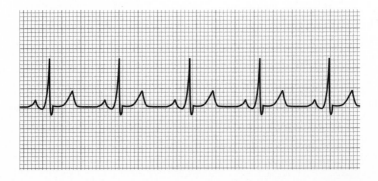

"You think it's muscular? Did it change when he moved? Well, then, you'd better ask."

I go to intermediate, then minor, write down some stories, let my other two colleagues go home to bed.

In minor, charts fall to the floor. I grab the clipboard of the next to be seen and work through the alphabet of rooms. A bug crawled into a man's ear. A young couple share a common cold. A lady dropped a wine glass and tried to pick it up, cutting—

Hiss. "Dr. Maskalyk, please call triage. Dr. Maskalyk, call triage." *Click.*

I look at the clock.

Three a.m. Bars closed. Probably a trauma.

"Excuse me, ma'am," I say, wrapping the bandage back around her finger.

I punch numbers into a wall phone.

"Triage."

"Hey. It's James."

"Oh, hi. We just got a call from an ambulance. Young male, facial smash. Unconscious. What else . . ."

"Intubated?"

"No. Scoop and run."

"ETA?"

"They said five minutes."

"Call the trauma team?"

"Done."

"You seen Ellen, my senior?"

"She was in major a few minutes ago."

"'Kay. Bye."

Hiss. "Could I have two nurses to trauma. Two nurses to the trauma room." *Click.*

I duck my head into the room I just left. "I'll be back in a little while," I lie.

I scribble an order for tetanus vaccine, set the chart down on the minor desk, and go to major. I pass through the waiting room. The prisoner is back in jail. Black eye, no damage to the globe. In his place, a drunk man lolls in a chair, legs akimbo, chin on his chest, snoring. Two young women sit beside each other, in black dresses and high heels. One has her head on the other's shoulder and a bag of ice at her wrist. She looks up as I hurry past. Mascara streaks her cheeks.

In major, nurses gather at the desk deciding whose turn it is to don one of the trauma room's heavy lead vests. I pick up a phone and page Ellen overhead. She steps from behind a closed curtain.

"What's up?"

She should have picked up that overhead page calling the nurses to trauma. I'll bring it up later.

"Trauma. Couple minutes away, facial smash, unconscious. Not intubated, which means they might have tried but didn't get it. Team's on the way. What are you thinking?"

"Possible difficult airway?"

"For sure. Probably full of blood. What do you want to get ready?"

Hiss. "Dr. Maskalyk to the trauma room." *Click.*

"Too late."

I pull some gloves off the wall and a plastic face shield from a cart. I hand them to her as we walk down the hallway towards the trauma bay. The doors wheeze open.

"Good luck," I say, and turn around.

I walk away from her, then out of the ER through the side door, to the ambulance bay, and outside.

Snow loops on the black pavement. An ambulance beeps as it backs quickly to our ramp, stops. A man leaps out, rushes to the back door, springs it open. In the back, another medic sits beside a stretcher, squeezing a bag. They push the bed from the truck's boxed back and two legs click down, two more, and they rush up the ramp.

I hurry beside them, pull my surgical gown tight against the wind. The man's face is swollen, his eyes just slits. Blood burbles out of his snoring mouth, spatters on the clear rubber mask. The trauma door opens, and I let the stretcher pass through, then hover, hidden by a curtain at the entrance. Ellen is at the head of the bed, Zainab beside her, a few feet back. The medic squeezes the bag and starts to recite the story breathlessly.

"Twenty-something male . . . assaulted . . . to the face and neck. Unwitnessed. Heart rate 120, sat 80 per cent, blood pressure . . ."

The room is full of nurses and residents looking at Ellen. She glances around for me.

I watch her sweat.

She intubates him. It is hard to stand back, but I manage. The surgery resident is beside the patient's neck, ready with the scalpel, plastic shield over his eyes. Zainab stands, riveted, eyes wide, three paces back.

While the man is getting his broken face imaged a floor above, another hiss overhead. A woman dancing on her balcony, drunk, high, daring fate, slipped. She arrives in the trauma room, her neck craned behind her in a dull stare, already dead. We tell her brother, an hour later, underneath white lights. He nods bravely. Behind him, his father strokes his daughter's hair, whispers loving words into her cold ear.

At 5 a.m., a woman comes to the nursing station where Ellen and I sit looking at the man's fractured face on a computer. Blood has seeped through her bandage. "I've been waiting for more than two hours, you know," she says, angrily, thrusts her wound at me.

"Well, ma'am," I say, "I'm the only doctor at night, and we see the sickest first."

Didn't you see the sign? Beside the palm tree?

So much misery in that one little finger.

A half-hour later: "Sorry for the wait. Let's see that hand." I carefully unwrap the gauze. "It'll come together nicely. There'll hardly be a scar."

She smiles, and in that square space, in the middle of the night, a bit of suffering disappears.

Saeed goes home, puffer in his pocket to add to the pile. The old man's brain shows no bright patch of blood, and I send him back to the nursing home with antibiotics for a urinary infection, death delayed another day. The man with the heart failure in bed 1 drops his oxygen when he walks, can't get the air past the water stuck in his chest, so I call cardiology. He'll be admitted until we can get more of it out. Thirty-six-year-old with chest pain goes home, the ache he held in his heart from great worry.

A suicidal woman changed her mind after the wine wore off. Couple of sprained ankles. A broken one. Nose-bleed. Two alcoholics slept in the hallway before stagger-ing out the door to go at it again. Miscarriage. Broken wrist. Back pain. Back pain. Chest pain. A man looking for a place to sleep out of the snow. A nurse from the ICU poked herself with a needle and is worried about HIV. I refuse a man opiates for his long-healed leg, and he storms out of the room, spilling orange juice on the ground. Never do see the one waving papers.

Six a.m. happens. I fight fatigue's familiar nausea. One by one, yawning residents disappear to their call rooms for an hour of sleep, and a plea for the ambulances to stay away.

The day's first workers walk through the hospital ("Morning . . . Morning . . ."). Zainab brings me a coffee. Sun starts to bleed black edges from the frosted windows, and with that, a faint but familiar echo of victory from the first time I made it through one of these.

I see my last patient in minor, review the man's broken face with the two students, pointing out the lines that don't connect to Zainab, asking Ellen what type of surgeon he would need and when.

"Plastic surgeon. A week or so. In case the breaks are visible. Aside from that, they'll heal. Does he need antibiotics?"

No. We talk about the shift. Zainab had one of the most exciting nights of her life. Ellen feels she could have handled the trauma a bit more smoothly, that it took her too long to decide about the airway. We get our one-sentence stories straight for the handover.

Cathy, my colleague, shows up, snow on her shoulders, puddles beneath her boots.

"Sorry I'm late . . . the roads."

"No troubles. Bed one, going to the morgue. Bed two . . ."

The two students and I linger near the ER's door, talk about a few last things for them to learn, patients we would follow up on.

"See you next time."

The door swings open.

Outside is bright, even with all the swirling snow. I leave my bike chained where it is and stamp my feet at the corner, waiting for a streetcar to scrape to a stop. People crush to its door then sit silent, headphones in, scrolling screens. I lurch in the aisle, scan faces, see age, sadness, sickness. A few quick glances meet mine, then back to their thoughts, everyone alone, a separate centre of a moving universe.

On my slippery street, storeowners roll up metal shutters, dust the sidewalk free of flakes. A woman walks past me, knocks me with her purse.

"Sorry!"

I'm at my desk, waiting for my mind to settle into the space my body is pointing to. My eyes swim with microsleeps and bits of dreams. I can't read, and it's tough to write, but I don't want to sleep. There's already so little time.

F is for flow.

F is for fucked.

I've gone into the same goddamn room twice to ask the same person a different question, and need to do it a third time. It's humiliating. Everyone is frustrated today. You can feel it.

"Are you kidding me?" a nurse says, glaring at a volunteer who sets down another four charts on the minor desk. The volunteer wilts.

The hospital is jammed. It's flu season, and a whole ward is closed for quarantine. Admitted patients crowd the hallways. Nurses are calling in sick.

I grab three more charts.

Over my shoulder, a nurse talks to me. "The first two sound like colds, and the guy in F, I have no idea why he's here. He told triage chest pain, but with me, he started to talk about his feet, and then he fell asleep."

"Great."

I duck into bed C for the third time.

"Sorry, I forgot to ask, have you travelled to any tropical countries?"

No.

"OK, I'll check that x-ray."

Will I? Maybe not. I duck back into the room.

"Actually, once it's done, find me, and I'll check it."

That's better.

With so many things to do, it's better to take things off my list than add them.

My flow is for shit today. Sometimes it's like that. Distracted, sick, thrown off by a mistake or someone yelling in your face, you never really land back fully into the middle of what you are doing. Today, though, the hospital's flow is stuck too. The two can go together. Once you learn what to do with a sickness, the work becomes handling five at a time, keeping the wave of humans moving through these beds and chairs.

The ER is in constant motion. People move through this space, sometimes smoothly, sometimes with difficulty, but no one stays.

"Hey, Jen. Can you throw an IV into that guy in B? He's dry. Start a litre, then you can move him to the chair."

"I'll add it to the list," she says, annoyed, puffing up a blood pressure cuff on an old woman's arm. "Ma'am, can you stay still?"

The guy in bed B is dehydrated. Vomiting, diarrhea.

I'm sure he'd rather stay in the room, but on a day like today . . . oh shit.

I turn around. "Actually, leave him in that room. He might be contagious."

She keeps staring at the jittering needle, and I turn away, lest she kill me.

Humiliating.

There are different kinds of flow. The ER's, the hospital's, the kind through our veins. As doctors, we are taught to pay particular attention to this last one. We call it different things as it moves through a body, blood or spinal fluid, the shifting sea that denies gravity, leaks back and forth, then out.

More than two litres of water passes through us each day, leaves in the fog of breath, from our skin and piss. On hot days the loss is greater, and with a fever even more. If you get sick with diarrhea, a bolus of bacteria survives your acid stomach to feast on the food in your intestine, their poisonous division loosens your tight junctions and water spills out. If it spills faster than you can put it in, you run dry, and die from all the salt left behind.

Change is ceaseless in the body too. Parts swap out for parts, get broken down, munched smaller, crafted into something else. Everything must move to create itself anew, and if there's not enough fluid in our vessels for a large slow pulse to push things around, we'll make fast small ones. Our heart races. Eighty. Ninety. One hundred. Hundred forty.

Uh-oh.

More than this, if we continue to bleed fluid, our beats run dry, pressure falls, and the shock starts. The process starts to fail. This is a last sign.

"I'm . . . so . . . cold."

With that sentence, trauma room nurses and ER doctors know they are a few deft moves away from a suddenly dead person.

The feeling is so close, I can touch it in my memory. The dread is unforgettable, and best shared, which is why you can't teach over a computer, or just send dollars. There's no chill in a spreadsheet with numbers of children dead from diarrhea or women who give birth and won't stop bleeding. You must put yourself in the middle of that troubled spot, wrestle with its questions while listening to the wails to know what's at stake. Otherwise it just seems a shame, and nothing lasting has ever been built on that.

Once, on a dry, blowing road between Nairobi and Somalia, I passed a convoy of tanks, artillery, and a hundred troops shielding their eyes from the sun and drifting sand. Behind me, half a million Somalis lived in tents. Beyond them, a vague border they had crossed with great loss. The troops were not stopping at the camp.

As the fighting worsened, people pinned now from both sides, more of them fled to Dadaab, the world's biggest refugee camp. Soon, the maternity room floor was full of labouring women, and the feeding centre bloomed thirsty children who'd walked weeks. On the road, there was little water, and when they arrived at the camp, unannounced, by the hundreds, there was little more, certainly not enough to clean their clothes or wash their bodies.

To plan water for hundreds who leave their houses with what they can carry, you need time to dig wells or truck in a minimum of 10 litres per person for cooking, cleaning, washing, drinking. The amount seems ample, even luxurious, until you learn that a single Canadian uses 300 litres a day. These 290 extra litres are shat into, dumped down drains, pushed through hops to make beer or tarry sand to grab oil. Soon, we will go to war over what water's left. Ethiopia is damming the Nile. Egypt and Sudan are anxious. Yemen's capital is running dry. Los Angeles too. The majority of Chinese wells are polluted. It is coming faster than we think.

With no fluid, an adult will die in about five days; children, faster than that. Some families were so dry when they arrived, they drank what was on the ground, sifting it through a piece of cloth, but it stayed dark and dirty, floating with bacteria.

In the hot sun, outside the feeding centre, on white plastic tables covered with white plastic sheeting, stretched a line of dehydrated children. Around the forearms of those too sick to swallow, nurses tied the rind of a rubber glove, and after a few seconds, the collapsed veins, trickling fluid towards the heart, would fatten enough to put a needle in. I could never get it, couldn't see the flat things, thin as a pencil lead under black skin, but the nurses, they rarely missed. Mothers would cluck-cluck-cluck as their children cried.

The intravenous catheter, the blood and water it delivers through its hub, has allowed for women to survive the bloodiest births, liquid to trickle into the desperately dry. A catheter twice the diameter of one the same length allows sixteen times the flow. It is a case of friction, and layers moving on layers. Asked again and again by my teachers about a treatment for an imaginary dying person, I repeated a phrase so often it became one word: "two large-bore IVs, running wide open."

We dripped salty water into these little kids, and some would live, others would die. A study came out around the same time, confirming what we'd learned from experience: that if you ran the water in too fast, it would flood the lungs of some, and they'd die gasping. It was just hard to tell them from the ones who needed it briskly.

F is for fucked.

"Doctor? The x-ray's done."

"Oh, right. I'll look at it."

The hospital is alive in its own way, perpetually changing, growing even. Movemovemove. The pressure pulls at me. After about two minutes of listening, an urgency sprouts, and my legs grow restless. I should be somewhere else. I interrupt.

Five minutes of listening can seem an eternity. Half an hour? Wow. Who knows. Doing CPR on a kid, that's different. There's nowhere else to be then.

Decisions are what keep things flowing in the ER and they must be made in the face of incessant interruptions from a growing list of evolving emergencies. It is rare to finish a thought without an x-ray technician saying, "Your patient can't sit up" or an overhead page suggesting the man you passed in the waiting room, bleeding and glaring, has lost what little shit he had left. Unless the interruption involves a sudden collapse of the first three letters of the alphabet, I've learned that it is best to finish what you've set out to accomplish, let the interrupters wait with their business until you finish with what's yours.

It takes effort to attend to a new object of focus, even more to return. You want your flow to be frictionless.

"OK, ma'am. I'll check it."

Patients come not in sequence as they do in books, but in bunches. If a person can wait hours, she's put in line, but if she can't, the line disappears, and there is just a list of shifting priorities.

Manage them. Once, a small boy arrived after chewing an electrical cord. He was screaming, and every single eye hurried to his side. Nurses with children of their own were keen to comfort him and the frantic mom. Cleaners stood, gaping, blue plastic carts forgotten. Even the registration clerk who had followed with the child's hospital bracelet waited outside the curtain, listening, fascinated. I too wanted to know how the story would go, but when I heard the cries, I was at the bed of an injured man who had hit a curb, then his handlebars with his belly, then the ground, who was now saying, despite being swaddled in blankets, how he felt so cold. On the other side of the wall, an ambulance had laid down a woman gasping for air. I'd seen a student nurse go in there twenty minutes before to start an IV and hadn't seen her come out. Her supervisor was next to the screaming child. That's the heat, the friction of layers of indecision and unfinished business.

With time, we learn to cut through it.

Pay attention, to every little thing. That's the main trick. This is no time for dreams.

The child was wailing, so it was not an "A" problem, at least not yet, and he was surrounded by help. The young, cold man, he was about to die, that was for sure.

He had seconds, or minutes, I couldn't tell which, so just presumed the worst. That's what good doctors do. It's why people tell stories about their mother, given two months to live, who survived for many. It's not because she met fools, but because it is wiser to prepare for the most precipitous outcome and be wrong about it.

The man was short of blood. Until he could get some, he needed salt water, as fast as possible, through two large-bore IVs wide open.

I told a porter to run, get some blood, from wherever was closest, didn't matter where. And a surgeon on the phone, I called after him.

Never delay a decision when you have enough information to make it, and always follow a decision as closely as possible with an action. If you don't, indecision and inaction multiply into chaos. Decisions create order. That's what this alphabet is about.

On the way to the child's cry, I glanced at the lady gasping from a failing heart. She was old, eighty. Failing hearts fall further and further behind, never really catch up. She was drowsy, counting down last breaths. An IV was finally in place, thank god. Minutes. I tapped a nurse at the foot of the child's bed, told him to draw up the drugs I needed for her intubation.

The boy was pushing gauze away from the corner of his mouth, still screaming, his face red. Someone handed me the phone. The surgeon was waiting in the OR. The porter clicked off the brakes of the injured man's bed, rolled the man to the elevator, blood running in fast through both IVs.

The boy's lips were oozing, not spurting. I asked the mom to apply pressure, promised to test his hemoglobin, and returned to the woman gasping in her room. New patients arrived. Charts piled.

Timelessness. It isn't always like this, so many sick people at once, or with decisions so clear, but when it is, hours disappear. No here or then, just one stretching moment, and when a replacement comes at the end of your shift, you can't believe it's already over.

The young man left the OR, his broken spleen cooling in a clear plastic bag. The woman with the failed heart rested on a ventilator, her heart beating easier with the work of breathing taken away. The little boy was calm, looking through a book filled with stickers. The blood had stopped with pressure, and he was waiting to be admitted until the clot became strong.

Correlates to this type of flow exist in modern psychology, and in antiquity. In the former, flow comes with complete immersion in a task—no actor, only action. Painting a picture, endlessly editing sentences, or making jumpshot after jumpshot until the buzzer sounds. Capacity meets purpose.

Taoists call it wu-wei, doing without doing, spontaneously and effortlessly rolling with what's moving. Resistance bleeds energy, and energy is the most precious thing, so if you rid yourself of as many blockages as possible, you are put where you are needed, again and again, right in the middle, as reliably as a stream falling down a mountain. When the distinctions between actions and decisions disappear, that becomes true flow, movement without effort. We are water, at least mostly, so act like it.

In the end, there is no way to save time, only good ways to spend it. Though seconds matter, if the schizophrenic man nods uncertainly at the follow-up appointment you've made, fuck everything else, you need to call his mother, and if she's not in, let it ring at the shelter. Or, rather, someone else does, because in those thirty seconds until someone hands you back the phone, you've looked again at the boy, breathing softly in his mother's lap.

"The x-ray's clear. Likely a virus. Your cough should get better, not worse, OK? If it does, we're never closed, you come back, and we'll check you out again."

It is removal of this last layer, that there is not any better way to be spending your time than helping others, that allows you to find the direction again. Even if the rest of your flow is terrible, and you leave work two hours late, you get to sleep happy.

I clatter my keys onto the kitchen counter.

Wow. That was a shit day.

I get a beer from the fridge, then turn my phone off, lie on my couch. The hum of traffic starts to pull apart into separate sounds. The whine of a siren crowds out the street's noise, then fades. The wall clicks and settles. A voice in the hall, laughing. Nothing stays still, not for a moment. I drowse.

Grab.

That guy. The vomiting guy. Fuck.

I turn my phone back on.

"Yeah, it's Maskalyk. Can I talk to Sam? Hey, man . . . Oh, you found him. Sorry. Don't know what was wrong with me. Yeah, stomach flu. If he can drink, he should be good to go. OK. Thanks, man. Hope it slows down. Good shift."

G is for ground.

I've been cutting down my shifts in the last few years so I can spend more time on Ethiopia. I work about ten a month now. It's just enough to keep my skills up. Fewer, and my fingers fumble.

When I graduated, I did twice as many. During those months, being in the ER was simpler than it has been since. My flow was natural, my hands steady, and my patients' faces grew as indistinct as the date or time. It was the hours outside of work that started to hurt. It is easy to ignore your own worries when there is a never-ending list of worse ones placed in front of you. My relationship failed. Friends fell away. Beauty too. I felt fine.

I wasn't. Fatigue caught up with me and I slowed down for a minute, looked around, wondered where everyone was.

If we in ER gather in community, it is to talk about how to resuscitate a baby, to poke needles into fake plastic necks, or to practise for poison-gas subway attacks. We don't practise joy, how to stay well in the face of all the sickness.

Doctor, Nurse, heal thyself.

Or not. Those who work in the ER burn out faster than any other type of physician. I'm not sure if it's the shifts or the long, steady glimpse of humans on their worst day.

I think most of us would say that it's not the sickest that affect us, that it is the minutes in contact with them when we feel most well used. In a macabre way, we hope for the next person to have something really wrong with them, but it is more rare than you'd imagine to see a critical patient in Toronto, even in the trauma room, someone whose system needs the order the alphabet can bring.

Most of the work here is in minor. ERs are open all hours, and since the service is free, people often come in early, instead of an hour too late. Sometimes there is nothing wrong with their bodies at all. There are so many measures in place to keep people well, or to catch them before they get too sick, I can go weeks without intubating someone. Worried minds, though, latch onto subtle sensations that magnify with attention, and lacking context, they line up to be reassured. The two populations, the sick and the worried, mix together, and separating them keeps us up all night.

Suffering souls, though, there is no shortage of them. They circle this place.

Some sleep right outside, on sidewalk grates, wrapped in blankets, waiting. One is splayed in the clothes he lives in, face pressed against the metal grille in a deep, drunk sleep. Every few minutes, a subway passes below the grates, and a rush of warm air flutters his shirt like a flag.

Businesswomen spin in and out of an office tower's revolving doors. They cross the street, eyes dancing between their phones and streetcar ruts, pretending not to notice the figure on the ground. Shoppers with bags from the Eaton Centre dangling from their arms lean into the road looking for taxis, jump out of the way of rushing cars.

A guy across the street notices the body. He glances at it, then at the hospital, makes a calculation that there must be no better street grate in the city, and moves on. Others step over him, as if he was downtown city furniture.

Within a few blocks of my ER, there are a dozen shelters for abused women and the homeless. There are health clinics for indigenous people, gay men and women, refugees, detox centres, beds for kids who've run away from home. On my way to work I pass them, pierced, dyed, smoking. Sometimes I'll see them in the ER, shyly pulling away a bandage from the cuts they made on their arms.

Seaton House, a men's shelter just up the street, holds more than five hundred. It has an infirmary for the old and the sick, a special floor where the most craven alcoholics are given brandy every hour, so they don't die on those grates. A patient told me that the floors are patrolled by gangs, and if you've a bag, they will pin your arms from behind and rifle through it, taking what pills or dollars there are.

"They call it Satan House."

He was new to Toronto, to big cities even. He sat on our bed, his bag empty and eyes wide.

"I can't go back there. Drugs. Bugs. Fights. Can I stay here? Just one night?"

Sorry, man. Here's a list of other shelters, a central access number, a sandwich, a prescription for the medicines you lost, a number for our social worker who can help you fill it, a bus token, a bandage for your foot. But I'm sorry, this ain't no hotel.

He held his backpack tight, under the sheets, shook his head, no fucking way. Security hoisted him from the bed, a guard on each arm, walked him down the hallway, out the door, into the night.

We give out clean needles, single-use vitamin C sachets so people can dissolve crack or black tar heroin in its acid instead of sharing lemon juice and scarring their veins. Some people come in just for sandwiches, or to use the phone. Others, to sit in a chair.

One of my colleagues rolled a man in a wheelchair out into a storm. The man had been pretending he couldn't walk, but when Jeff's back was turned, he would stand, grab hand sanitizer from the wall, and drink it down. He'd been doing it for hours before someone noticed. After Jeff pushed the man out, he sat back down at the desk in minor, began angrily filling out the man's chart, paused, then slammed his pen down and, furious, snowflakes melting on his scrubs, wheeled the man back in. Our trust gets broken and broken and broken and broken, but underneath it is an even deeper caring.

A few years ago, I heard an overhead page—"Dr. Maskalyk to triage"—and I walked out, to help decide which way to direct a stretcher I'd guessed, and instead saw a bailiff who touched me with an affidavit, dropped it, furled, on the ground.

"Sorry," the registration clerk said to me, bashfully. "I thought he was a friend."

I picked up the rolled paper. A lawsuit. It named many doctors. I couldn't remember the complainant.

I got his chart from medical records. It didn't cue me. I'd met him once, two years before. I could remember the night. So busy, running from minor to major every few minutes. I have a vague memory of his back, but not his face.

The chart was mostly empty. "Flank pain" was his complaint, and I scratched in only a few physical findings. In the margin was a note from the nurse: "Verbal order, Maskalyk, morphine 5 mg IV." You get calls like that all the time, from a worried nurse, asking for pain relief for someone writhing in a stretcher. Sure, sure, I would have said, after I asked a few questions, 5 milligrams.

In the years that had passed, I had touched a hundred backs, seen many people in pain. This man was fine. There was no bad outcome. He had CT scans, MRIs, all negative. His charge to me was that I contributed to his opiate addiction. He named every doctor who had crossed his path.

The case dragged on for years. My lawyers kept telling me that it would go no further, but it kept limping. Every few months, another letter, until whoever was helping that man exhausted what money he had and the case was dropped.

Some of my colleagues haven't been so lucky. Sometimes that person with back pain that sounded the same as the hundred before in fact has a hemorrhage, or an infection, and becomes paralyzed. I received an angry letter from a family doctor who said I was incompetent for not x-raying the leg of a young woman he had sent to the ER. She hadn't fallen, hadn't endured an injury. I examined her leg. No swelling, no chance of a break. Not blue, good pulse. No emergency as far as I could tell. Does it hurt when you do this? Stop doing that, I said, every doctor's favourite piece of advice. Rest it, see if it gets better. It didn't. The bone had a tumour in it.

Shoulder pain in a drunk man, sleeping it off in the hallway. This time, I got an x-ray. Negative. The pain persisted. I CAT-scanned his neck. Broken. The pain was from a pinched nerve. He hadn't complained of neck pain, couldn't remember falling. But I didn't feel along his neck until much later. I should have. I didn't even put a collar on before I sent him to scan. A screaming radiologist called me in minor. "What the hell are you doing sending him up alone?"

First shift, after I graduated. A pharmacy student with severe asthma. Often, patients with chronic disease know what they need. Adrenalin, intramuscular, he said, requesting our most powerful drug. I found a nurse, told her what I wanted, stepped away to write on his chart, turned back to see the colour drain from her face, watched him fall back onto the bed. How did you give that adrenalin? I shouted, my finger already on his neck. Intravenous, she said, knowing her mistake, that in a living person, it must never go straight into the blood, that it is too much for a beating heart to take.

Shit, I said, lacing my fingers together before hammering down on his chest.

He lived. I told him what had happened, then my chief and the nursing supervisor. The patient understood, probably better than anyone in the world. At least my asthma's gone, he said, wincing as he tried to sit up.

I could go on. No matter how careful I try to be, I make mistakes. The next one is just waiting.

We are taught all kinds of things as we work our way down the alphabet. To spot a hurt person, to remain suspicious, to learn from our errors. It can be difficult to rest from the worry.

"You will fucking too see this patient," I said to a resident who refused to assess a woman with AIDS who couldn't stop vomiting long enough to take her pills and had nowhere to go. "Because it's your fucking job, that's why." Anger shook me.

"You stupid jew cunt!" a patient yells at my colleague.

"Handshandshands!" a security guard shouts as the man they are watching undress pulls a knife.

"I have hep C, and if any of you come close, I'll spit in your eye!" another man, scratched and bruised, screams, five cops holding him down. He was released from prison a day before, having served twenty for murder. In his hours of freedom, he beat another man nearly to death. "Come here," he says, looking at a nurse behind me. "I dare you."

I'll sue you. I'll stab you. I'll come back with a gun and kill all of you. You're a shitty doctor. You're an ugly nurse. You're an idiot. Goof. I want a second opinion. I want to kill myself.

Dying person, dead person. Sick person. Lying person. Faking. Manipulative. Poisoned. Raped. Dead.

Screaming. Crying. Writhing in pain. Hopeless. Afraid. Confused. Alone.

Wow, must be stressful, people say.

You get used to it, we answer.

Ground floor, downtown, ground down. Suffering can be contagious, and no matter the job you do, it just keeps coming back.

Your world view skews. If you don't make an effort to balance it, the ER becomes your new normal. Like a home, you turn to it for what you need. Your colleagues seem like the normal ones, because they can joke while a man, shot dead, lies behind them.

Daddy, a colleague's daughter said, all you do is work, sleep, and drink. A nurse told me after a string of five days in a row, she took a bottle of wine to bed, and cried.

It's hard to make it ten years here. Some don't make it two. It's worse for the nurses. They spend more time at the bedside, unobserved, unprotected. They watch people die over hours, asking, "Am I going to make it?" again and again. I get asked once. "We'll do what we can," I say, and move on.

The ones that last are changed. The shifts, the swearing, the shouts of pain, the anxiety and sadness and anger pouring from strangers. Miss a decimal place and someone's dead. Drug seekers lie to your face so they can flip pills on the street, and you grow suspicious of those in real pain. The addicts and alcoholics who circle this place, lost and dying, whom you can't help and no one else wants. A security guard had his nose broken one week. A nurse, a chunk of hair ripped from her head. She waited until it stopped bleeding, then finished her shift. I haven't seen her since.

We work when we are sick, masks over our faces so we're not contagious. I broke my arm, and didn't miss a day. We have a silent agreement to not ask for help. Sickness becomes weakness, weakness a sickness.

It's rare to connect with the people I treat. The ones I do best for wake up in the ICU, in a sedative haze, not sure what happened or whom to thank. We deliver more dead babies than live ones. No one shouts, "Mazel tov! It's appendicitis!"

We don't develop relationships with patients, claim that we prefer it that way. We dive deep, straight, unapologetically, unsentimentally, into a person's worst fears, ask them about sex, drugs, who's hurting them, why they're hurting themselves. We look in their eyes, watch them cry, put needles into their veins until they're plump with water, dab blood from their cervixes, know their bodies more intimately than they ever will. When the new shift comes in, we go home and try to live in ours.

I sat in my first suit, tugging at the cuffs, and told the doctors across the table, ones who were deciding whether they would let me into their emergency training program, that I thrived on the type of challenges the ER presented. I didn't mind odd hours and had healthy habits to make up for tough nights. They nodded, satisfied, and I walked out, past a half-dozen nervous young men and women, their answers the same as mine.

We get ground down anyhow. The pace, we'll say, images of mangled limbs we take with us wherever we go. It's hard to leave, even if you know you should. It feels good to be surrounded by those who know what you do, to whom you don't have to explain.

Some of us make it through. Some drink. Some smoke. The ones who last best, laugh. Even about the black things. Especially about the black things. Without the absurd, there is only tragedy.

A woman, twenty, fell down twenty stairs. One eye was swollen shut. She wouldn't answer to her name or open her other eye. She pushed at the nurse's hands that tried to help her, again and again, sought to climb out of bed. I sedated her until she was still, and did a CAT scan of her brain. The scan showed bruising, blood in the grey matter where there should be none, a slick of it pooling inside her skull, squeezing her brain tighter and tighter. I called the neurosurgeon, a German, and explained what I saw.

"So she needs the OR," I said over the phone.

"Is she . . . pretty?" he said in a heavy accent, chewing, swallowing.

"I don't know . . . I guess so."

"Zen we must to do everysing," he said, and hung up the phone.

A few hours later, nurses and I recalled the conversation as we switched back and forth for CPR. We laughed, above an old woman's still heart, caught ourselves, turned our eyes back to our work, and fell into smiles.

You can see those who are edging out. When we're unable to meet the sadness, or to laugh about it, cynicism takes hold. Even worse, anger. We curse nurses on other floors for being too slow. We criticize our colleagues' decisions, their flow, their bad day, forgetting that they, like us, are just trying to make it through a shift, a week, a month, a life, surrounded by all the pain.

Last, we curse our patients. This is a final sign. Touching many people, but being touched by none of them, they close like a flower that no longer sees the sun. It's as if every person takes away from you something you need.

Not her again, a nurse says under his breath, as a volunteer places a chart of a regular on the desk, as if this wasn't the point of the place, as if this didn't happen twenty times a day.

People think that to make it through, we become inured, develop some kind of barrier, beyond emotion. It doesn't work like that. You can offer an illusion of indifference, even tell yourself that you've got it handled, but all that tough stuff makes it in just the same. What shuts down is the part that turns it around.

There's too much to do, a next patient to see, and if you're never told how important it is to work on anger and fear as it comes up, you put it off, and the frustration diffuses into all aspects of your being, its origins almost invisible. You can get so behind, you abandon the project. Then, on that fateful day, when you have a chance to do something right for someone you don't know, or cut a corner, you say to yourself, "Fuck it."

The end has come. Time to quit.

People do. Plenty. I'll see them in the hall after many months, when I used to see them every day. Miss us? I'll ask. Yeah, they say, I do, some of them wistful. But I just couldn't do it anymore. It wasn't good for me.

What they mean is, instead of just the worries following them home, some numbness did too. Joy started to seem for fools, because while there are many things we will never know, what we do know for certain is that one day, a bullet meant for someone else will whip through our body, our foot will turn on a dog's toy on the second stair and we will fall, or a cough will tickle our chest then sputter a tablespoon of blood, and in an instant we know what it means.

It's here.

H is for hurt.

Sirens cut through the glass.

My clock is upside down. I got home at four this morning, slept for a few hours, woke early to take my visa to the embassy and to do the many things one must before being away for months. Cancel memberships, cut a set of keys for my friend, Mark, finish my hospital charts, throw a party.

It's one of the reasons I picked the ER, and its night shifts. My days are completely free: no patient practice, no one to disappoint when I'm away. I don't need a secretary, or office chairs, just a place to hang my jacket, and once I have handed over unfinished business to a colleague, I walk out into the snow, leave the work behind.

Or that's what I say. The heart, though, doesn't cleave things so neatly as the mind.

That last shift in minor—the one where I wanted to go home so badly I forgot the vomiting man, nauseous and alone in his room—as I was stacking up my charts, a woman came to the counter, frustrated from the wait, son shrinking behind her, and asked in an angry voice, "How much longer are you going to make us wait? My son's coach told us he might have a concussion, and he should be seen right away. It's one in the morning!"

Wrong day for this, lady.

We pounced on her. Me. The clerk. Nurses.

"Ma'am, take a look around . . . Two hundred and fifty patients today . . . in the order they come . . . some very ill people . . . you're free to leave . . . could be another two hours . . ."

"Well then, we're just going to go to another hospital!"

"Can't recommend it. It's no prison. Sure. Sign here. Up to you . . ."

She left, "against medical advice," even though that's what we were advising. Her son, at this point, was hidden around the corner, head retreating into his parka like a turtle. We could all tell he was OK. After they walked out, a few of us shook our heads, like, "Some people . . . ," but we knew we had got it wrong.

How to not help others, and hurt yourself? Easiest thing in the world. Don't see them. Don't recognize their hurt, because you can't see past your own.

You must be very worried. We can tell you love him very much. He'll be OK. We'll get to him as quickly as we can, just a few more people ahead. Sorry for the long wait. It gets to us too.

So simple. I get relief just writing the words. They

would have helped us all remember why we were there, if one of us had had the wisdom to say them.

No one did, though. Mistakes in the ER are not only about giving the wrong person the wrong drug. They're about letting what you're carrying stand in the way of helping others.

We get caught up in parts of bodies. Ankles on a flat screen, manic minds spinning nonsense. We pull people into smaller and smaller parts until maybe there's nothing but a straggling uric acid pair on a strand of DNA, when right there, blinking at you, telling you that the problem is bigger than a sickled cell, she's missing school nearly every week, can't concentrate from the pain and her grades are suffering, is a whole human being. Despite all our advances, it remains the basic unit of the work, though fewer and fewer people are experts in it.

Here's a doctor's note, follow up with your hematologist, we say, as if that doctor might help with her marks.

In medical school, we're not taught that it's as important to take care of ourselves as it is others, that if we don't, we're living in defiance of what we hope to deliver. We get some vague words, maybe a weekend on wellness, but we're never really asked to understand that we should be well in as many ways that matter, not just so we stay fit next to sickness but so we know the direction of being truly healthy.

I don't think my teachers were keeping it a secret, just that they didn't know this themselves. It was a private recipe that some knew through grace and error and others abandoned completely, becoming one of those doctors who lived in the hospital, rolled through husbands, and made enough money to have a wing named after them until a richer person pried the plaque off.

By residency, when we were supposed to learn everything that mattered, it was too late to care. The hours were crushing. We rushed through the stream of rotations, our pagers rarely quiet. Friends questioned the wisdom of being made to work so many hours in a row, but it was always clear to me. We were given the opportunity, again and again, to be lost to the work, as ready as a platelet. If healing was the point of this place, it wasn't for us.

I bought it. It was the encouragement I was waiting for. How lost could I get? All the way so I never had to come back? There was a whole world of despair to sink into, where mine would just disappear like a wave in its ocean.

I found Médecins Sans Frontières. I thought it would be a challenge, and by facing it, I might find something to soothe me. A new knowledge. An accolade. A community that helped reconcile the injustice I had seen. A mission to save the world, and with it, myself.

I had no idea. I thought I was prepared, that I had enough willpower to churn through whatever I was faced with. I would eat the suffering, metabolize it as if it was my superpower, like I had done the pain from my own past. I hadn't, of course. I had only arranged a life where I didn't have to face it.

I talked with a close friend as I stepped onto the plane. Why are you going, man?

Because I want to see who I am when everything is taken away.

I did.

Hurt.

Couldn't hide behind the violence, nor the sickness, nor my patients.

It wasn't just that it was harder than I expected, which it was, but I wasn't who I expected. I had what it took to get me in there. The enthusiasm, the skills. I just didn't have what I needed to make it out OK. You know how I know? I left a little girl there, Ayen Juk Ring, whom I started to love, and I didn't even cry, just put up another wall. My poor heart. I lied to it every day.

I cry for her now. Finally, perhaps, I am learning. I've emailed friends in Abyei, but over the years, more and more have left. I've come close a few times. Last I heard, she may have been in Tonj, South Sudan. The trail has grown dim.

I read the stories of women and girls raped and killed, others left to suffocate in shipping containers, the war much worse than it was when I was there. It's possible trying wouldn't have made a difference, but I fear what not trying has allowed.

The Red Cross says they can't help. I look at photos of South Sudanese children in Ethiopian refugee camps who have lost their families. War is stamped on their faces. There's one photo I return to again and again. It's not Ayen, I'm sure, though it is a girl her age. But that's not why I look at it. It's because she's smiling. After all that.

I came back from the field in misery, and returned to the ER to make some money, so I could keep running. The book I promised to write about Sudan stopped me from doing that. Months before it was due to come out, a friend asked me how I would remember, in the brief but bright spotlight of attention that was due to swing my way, why I went in the first place. I had not considered the question. I knew she was a wise person. She once asked me if I had found romance, and I said I wasn't yet ready to have someone's happiness depend on me. She answered, "Well, James, some people won't get a dog because they're afraid to watch them die. What a small life they have."

I didn't want to leave the work, but I needed to do it from a different place, one that didn't make me so sick. I needed to stay close to the ground, so I did it in the most literal way I could think of: I sat on it. I rekindled what I remembered from a meditation practice I left years before, started counting my breaths. As it goes, a teacher appeared, taught me to untangle my experience, and I joined him for silent weeks. Know what makes you, he said.

I did more MSF, this time in Kenya, in that refugee camp I told you about. Until I learned I was going to live there, I had never heard of the sprawling complex, though it was the fastest-growing city on the planet.

I woke up each day with the call to prayer and the soft knocks on my neighbours' doors, my Muslim friends saying in Somali, "Brother, time to pray." As they shuffled towards the mosque, I would roll from my mosquito net, sweep the sand from my floor, and sit, saying my own prayers for that day.

The truck would gather us, and we would swish over the shifting ground towards the feeding centre, where I learned to mourn, then take us back to our gated enclosure, where I learned to find joy when I could. After five months, I left for Ethiopia, and arrived well, happy, no sick memories, just sad ones about the great work that remained. I understood that the best promise I could make to all the hurting people was to not add another.

More teachers appeared. A man I first met deep in the woods. I asked him if he wanted some coffee, and he paused, then said, "OK, but I don't usually take intoxicants. This," he said, gesturing to the wildness around us, "is usually enough." A woman who taught me the difference between will and willpower, that the latter gets tired from all the pushing, that the former, born from deep within, beyond trying, would do the pushing for me. "Now that you are knowing yourself," she said, "you must learn to love what you find."

A physician, many years my senior, no longer practising, reminded me that the hurt was there not to be overcome, but so I would know what needed to heal.

Teachers were everywhere. A colleague at work, who never said a bad word about anyone, was always quick to laugh, would switch her shifts without my even needing to explain why. Another, who followed his patients, even called them at home the next day. Aklilu, two daughters of his own, driving two hours each day to get to Black Lion and work on a project that didn't pay in dollars and would long outlast him. A woman in a red scarf, exhausted and worried, her son hiding behind her, buried in his parka. My grandfather, quiet, patient.

All those years, and all those miles, looking in different places for who I was, when what mattered was *how*.

Can you make dragging someone from his bed, his backpack in a plastic bag because of all the bugs, out into the snow an act of love?

Yes. That's the practice.

I unclipped earrings from the lobes of an old woman, hit crossing the road, before she was moved through the spinning ring of the CT scanner so the x-rays would not be dazzled by the metal. I put them in a clear plastic bag. With the first few cuts of the scan, I could tell the earrings were never going back on.

"Isn't it strange," I said to my colleague, after I rode the elevator down, "to take out someone's earrings for the last time."

"I don't even think about that, man."

You will.

A Tibetan boy with a painful rash. I did what I learned in Dadaab, acted as though his father wasn't there, introduced myself, sat with my face at his height, at a comfortable distance away, looked him in the eye and smiled. We talked about his shirt, the weather, what was happening in school these days. Then we came to the rash. I lifted his shirt gently. It was chicken pox that he had scratched into a painful bacterial infection. Antibiotic cream would clear it quickly. I reassured him and left the room. I was at the desk writing a prescription when his father came up to me and said:

"There is a healing that can happen without even touching someone. You did that for my son. His pain is better already. Thank you."

Tears filled my eyes. I got it. I felt rejuvenated. The medicine helped me too.

The man who was hurt the other night, the one with the smashed face, is in the ICU. I went to visit him today. He still hasn't woken up fully. His eyes are taped shut, his hands wrapped in gauze and tied to the bed, because when the sedation wears thin, he'll grab at what's near, pull out his IV lines, or worse, the endotracheal tube he needs to keep his airway open.

His mother was there, knitting, waiting. I introduced myself, and we shook hands solemnly.

Do you mind if I sit with you?

No.

It took her a minute, but she started to talk. He worked downtown, at two jobs. He had a five-year-old daughter he loved and who lived with her mom. He was working double time to help her out.

I listened for a while longer, then stood.

He'll be well taken care of here.

She nodded.

We shook hands again, and I left.

I is for images.

Past the swinging doors of the ambulance ramp and around the triage window. The security guard stands up. I take off my hat. He recognizes me and sits back down.

"You looked like a mental patient," he teases.

"Give me a few more years."

"Ha ha. Me too," he says, puts his feet up, and his eyes shift back to the screens.

I grab a thick folder with my name on it, stacked with half-filled charts. When it's busy, I write just a few words to help me recall the story of an arm, or a headache. We all do it. Saves us minutes.

"Hi, Dr. Maskalyk," one of the clerks says to me, facing away, studying a man's health card.

"Hi, Janelle," I say, closing the door softly behind me.

Insulated by these heavy metal doors, I don't see what she does. I miss the worry on the face of a husband, craning his neck, trying to catch a glimpse of his wife bundled into blankets, her health card in his hand, people selling drugs to waiting patients, others falling in love. My circle is small.

I pass the major desk. Natalie is leaning against it, holding a chart.

"Well look who it is. Dr. What's-His-Name. Are you here to work or just to walk around?"

"Supervise. At the last department meeting, I don't think you were there, we decided that whenever you're on, we should have a second doctor nearby."

"As a matter of fact, I *was* at that meeting, because it was my turn to do rounds, and I distinctly remember you weren't there."

"My aunt died again."

"How many times is that now?"

"It's eleven times."

"Eleven. That's a lot."

"It just doesn't get any easier."

"Funny."

"No, charts. Off to Addis in a few days."

"Didn't you just get back?"

"Seems like it. Some people are going for drinks tomorrow. You working?"

"Oh yes. Got me a hot date with intermediate."

"Well, come after, if you want."

"You know me. I'm always stuck here forever. But I'll try."

"All right. I'm just around the corner if you need to run anything past me."

"I'm so lucky."

I clear half-full cups and prescription carbons from a section of desk, set the folder down. It is thick with people, the worries and numbers that make them. Well, a single image, a snapshot of a person and their life. I turn over the first. My illegible scrawl.

36M. Detox request. Belt. Waiting room. Code white.

Last month, Janelle's voice on an overhead page, cool, almost bored. "Code white, waiting room. Code white, waiting room."

Code white, an agitated person. The nearest doctor attends, determines whether the person is well enough to be pushed from the hospital, down the ambulance ramp, back onto the street, told they can come back when they're calm.

I punched the metal button and the intermediate doors swung open to the waiting room. At the registration desk, Janelle stood, arms folded, curious, looking towards the rows of chairs.

A man waiting for a medical clearance for detox was picking fights. The others in the waiting room crowded away from him, some standing, nervously glancing to where he sat. He was short, with a tattooed neck, knee bumping up and down. I arrived at the same time as our security guards, and as we approached him, he stood, calmly removed his shirt, unloosed his belt, heavy with metal brackets, and started swinging it in circles in front of him, like a cowboy with a lasso trick.

"Come on," he said, tongue pink behind his missing front teeth.

Four security guards in black padded vests glanced at me.

"Time to go outside, brother."

They slowly circled him.

I write more. *Alert. No apparent injury. Escorted out by security.*

Like they were going to a dance.

47M. Jaundice. Ascites. Liver failure. Actor.

A handsome yellow man, his belly pregnant with fluid from a failed liver, and a piece of gauze shoved in his nose to stanch bleeding his liver couldn't stop anymore.

"Hey, Doc. Take a few litres off of me?"

I showed a medical student how to pierce through his skin with a hollow needle, attach it to a tube. Yellow fluid that had drifted through vessel walls, no proteins to provide a counterargument, spilled into a bottle on the floor. We drew five litres from abdomen.

"I can move again!" he said, pushed himself off from his elbows to the side of the bed, fluid dribbling from the hole we made.

"Wait, wait. We'll get you a Band-Aid."

He winked at us.

I turn over some more pages, add a few words, sentences, evidence for the courts, to my colleagues that I did what I could to help.

71M. No fixed address. Found in subway. Intoxicated. No injury.

Can't place this face. Maybe I didn't even see it, covered, snoring in the hallway.

I turn over the nursing note. Empty.

The invisible man.

30F. Hearing loss. Traumatic. Abuse. Counselled. Refused.

A bloody eardrum, purple and bulging, the man who did it pacing outside the door, afraid to leave me and his wife alone. She didn't tell the triage nurse, or even me at first. I guessed. Let me call the police, I said. He'll do it again. He doesn't love you. He wants to kill you. He will do it. I'll get our security guards. Have you seen them? They're fucking huge. You'll be safe. We'll find a place for you to stay.

She shook her head.

Will my hearing come back?

Tough to say.

What?

TOUGH TO SAY, I repeated into her good ear.

61M. Back pain. Mechanical.

57F. Headache. Classic migraine. Metoclopramide.

24F. Tooth pain. Drug seeking.

29M. Diplopia. New father.

Double vision. A young father, red face under red hair, eyes tired but dancing. Upstairs, only a few hours earlier, his wife had given birth to his first child. A girl! And today was his birthday! Everyone's birthday, I said, laughing. His new family was sleeping, cuddled upstairs, but he was too excited, didn't want to go home, wouldn't be able to sleep if he did. Really, he said, I'm just wandering around the hospital, and I know I should be seeing my family doctor about this, sorry to bother you, but I'm seeing double.

No, you're not, I thought, and peered through to the black backs of his eyes. The flat disc of his optic nerve and the vessels that sprouted from it were fat with pressure.

Shit.

"I think we should get a CT scan."

"What do you think it is?"

It's bad, man. "Don't know yet."

I add: *Astrocytoma. Neurosurgery.*

Birthday, deathday.

I turn another over.

Another.

Weeks' worth of people, dozens and dozens. Recent ones I remember well, these older ones, though, the images are blurred, vague, and I just write what I always do. Some, though, erupt from my memory, there forever, vivid, unforgettable.

3 months M. Inconsolable infant.

A mother holding her wailing baby. When she put him down, he yelled even louder, and I heard a broken rib click. I couldn't believe it. I took x-rays. Broken legs too.

"Ma'am, I've got to ask you to leave the room." Behind me, security guard, social services, ready to take the crying boy.

How the fuck do you do that.

I need a drink.

I turn over another. *Headache. Prescription request.*

37F. Sexual assault.

Call the police, I said again, to a woman clutching her purse. No, she said, I've done that before. They make you go to court, bring out all of your sexual history, try to make it seem like you were asking for it. Just give me the morning-after pill, so I don't get pregnant.

Don't go, she said to the nurse. I don't want to be alone.

22F. Trauma.

Young woman, leg torn off at the thigh, white and dead on the trauma room stretcher, her friend from the same car accident in the next one, calling her name. The doors swing open, and I catch a glimpse of her mom and dad, frantic, talking to a police officer, waiting for news.

37M. Cocaine intox. Paranoid.

A man who smoked so much cocaine, he saw familiar faces in strangers, approached them and was shoved away. He heard people talking about him. While I was in the room, his eyes kept darting over my shoulder.

"You're sure they're not saying anything?"

When I asked the psychiatry resident to talk with him, she rolled her eyes.

I close mine.

Bright flashes of disappearing light. Stuttering images of a chart, and around the edges, a black screen on which bright purple pixels buzz and scatter.

A friend's plastic shoe in a puddle of blood, shining on the resuscitation room's shining floor. Alaina laughing, ducking, pushing, play fighting, green trauma gown wrapped at her waist. Security guard sheened with sweat, holding down a schizophrenic man, saving my life, risking his. Big yellow numbers of blood pressure. A man's face burned black, looking at me with wide, scared eyes and smoky glasses. Ellen bent over the smashed man's airway in the trauma room.

In Ethiopia, a cupboard covered in tape, nurses at the one white desk, papers scattered like leaves. Cement floors wet with chlorine, a man swirling it in circles.

Some images are tethered to sounds, some to feelings that tug at my chest, my face. Beyond the yellow blood pressure numbers, and Ellen bent all wrong over the airway, an urge to push her aside.

I open my eyes.

The chart of a bald blind man who had scratched his arms and legs so often they were thick with nail tracks. A woman with a jar full of invisible bugs. "Can you see them? They're right there." A Muslim man with a hernia, years of deep bows coloured on his forehead. A woman jerking in her light crack sleep, tissues falling from her bra.

I sign her chart, my last one. A stack of flat pictures of people who pass through this place. One day you, everyone you know.

I sit back, rub my face with my hands, yawn.

Hiwot's hopeful eyes as we pushed up and down on the chest of a young taxi driver. Birds circling in Addis Ababa's high sky, and the ground being eaten up by my black shoes.

J is for jubilee.

Ugh.

Light has crept around the corner of my blackout screen.

Daytime.

I turn to my side, listen. It's quiet.

I roll towards my side table, fish for my phone in the dark, blink it on.

Ten, I'm hoping for ten.

Noon. Shit.

I roll out of bed, click the lamp on. My mirrored closet shines back at me. My eyes are red and narrow, the lines on my face drawn sharply.

I've been poisoned. By myself.

My mouth feels wrinkled on the inside. A familiar

ache in my sinuses, between my eyes. Nausea washes to the back of my throat.

The coming-home jubilee has dovetailed sweetly into a going-away one. These last years, it's tough to tease the two apart.

I count the drinks I had.

". . . four . . . five . . . jesus . . . six . . . *seven.*"

I curse myself, for the hundredth time, forgetting that what I look for in drink is an escape from the anxious voice of recrimination to whom everything matters.

I stand, steady, take a few steps to the bathroom, turn on the shower, find a wafer of ondansetron below the sink, and let it dissolve in my mouth. It's a serotonin antagonist, stops receptors in the stomach from passing on the pain. Someone once told me it gave her mood a boost, so now I believe it too. Mood is like that, waiting to be fooled, by drugs and words.

The mirror fogs. I drink a glass of water, then step into the shower. The steam wraps me like a blanket.

There are a few rules when supporting oneself through a season like this, particularly as it has lasted a couple of decades. First, the best thing for hangovers is to not have them. This advice, at least to this point, has been unrealistic.

In the true spirit of science, disproving hypotheses, I have discovered only two true cures. The first is to have no booze. The second is to have more booze. I can't recommend this last option. I've seen it go sour a hundred times. It has at the end of it, not just the shakes, but space on a street grate, and the quiet rebellion of your liver, one of the most loving parts of your body until the day it gives up, and you turn yellow, drowse, bleed, and die.

Aside from these two approaches, the task becomes one of hangover mitigiation, a worthwhile branch of science, despite its limited successes. In this study, it is best to space them out as far as possible. It allows a full experience of the sickness you've brought yourself, and after it's finished, lets you touch what it's like to feel completely well so you know what you're missing. If you don't, it's like smoking; you just get accustomed to feeling ill.

A caution. Though you may have stored in your memory a glorious night when you were twenty and went to bed after partying, to wake up after only a few hours' sleep feeling well and rested, this will never happen again. When you wake up in the morning feeling OK, it is because you are still slightly drunk. The worst is yet to come.

Here it is. I lean my head against the slick tiles.

I've made some important discoveries in the field, many of them borrowed, all of them difficult to remember when needed most. Drink only clear, not sweet things. A friend of mine taught me this. She would drink dry white wine, neither sweet nor red; vodka, not whisky; white rum, not dark; club soda, not cola. As such, the best drink to diminish hangover intensity is vodka and club soda in a pint glass. It is clear, neither delicious nor refreshing, and the bubbles prevent you from guzzling.

Beer from taps is best avoided. My friend Jehan, on his first shift as a barkeep in London, was stopped as he went to pour into the sink the beer that had collected under the tap's grate. We don't do that, he was told. Pour it back into the keg. Wow. OK. Which one, lager or ale? Doesn't matter.

In preparation for the morning after, prior to bed, I took a twenty-four-hour antihistamine, a dose of N-acetyl cysteine, and a milligram of melatonin. The hope with the antihistamine was to block one of the products found in wine that leads to the dilating throb of a headache. N-acetyl cysteine is a drug I use in the ER to protect the liver after someone downs a bottle of Tylenol, the surest way to die the worst death. There's no science behind my using it for alcohol, but let's face it, there's not a lot of science behind a lot of science. The melatonin helps me claim sleep that would otherwise be lost to tossing and turning. My Chinese doctor told me to take it every day for the rest of my life because, he says, I'm too old to make it on my own anymore. Shit.

Sometime around five, I woke up anyway. It's common. Once the alcohol level drops, the toxic metabolites, the poisons, and the exciting chemicals that have been released to fight alcohol's sedation circle in our blood. Eventually, we drop unconscious, but never touch the blackest, most healing sleep.

I drank a glass filled with fizzing sweet vitamin C and magnesium, swallowed an ibuprofen, lay back down. Taking painkillers before bed is for amateurs; they will have worn off by morning. Tylenol is not good here. It's metabolized by the liver, its cells already working overtime trying to chew up alcohol. The sugar prevents my glucose from falling while the liver is busy chewing up the wine.

The glass door steams. The ondansetron starts to work, and the tightness in my stomach uncurls. Or so I imagine.

As my patients try to teach me every day, there's only so many times you can do this to yourself, hurt a body that is trying to care for you. I started drinking at thirteen. Rum and root beer. The world spun. It still thrills.

What gets you? The booze, or never discovering what exactly you're trying to cover up?

The water starts to cool. I turn off the faucet. The pressure bangs pipes behind the walls of my small apartment. Tat-Tat-Tat.

I step from the shower. On the rack, where it always hangs, is my travel kit, with earplugs, medicines, toothbrush. I take a towel, clean steam from the mirror so I can shave.

The melatonin is keeping me bleary. Two more steps. A cup of black coffee, to obscure some of the sleep debt and constrict the blood vessels in my brain, keep the headache low. Then a run, get blood to every little part where the acetaldehyde is hanging on.

This is becoming like a part-time job. Harder livers through chemistry. Jolt the body awake with coffee, knock it out with wine, keep it down with drugs. Repeat.

Intoxicants are always close at hand to dull sharp edges. With them, familiar moments can seem new, full of insights and ideas, that fizzle short of action. They soften hard feelings, and even if booze or drugs don't turn you into the person you want, they make it feel, at least temporarily, as though the person you are is far away.

With enough practice, the flight becomes a life. The almost invisible line between a real moment and a less painful version of it blurs, and the feeling of release can seem nearly as good as the real thing. Soon, it's just what we reach for. In celebration, in sorrow, as reward, eventually, as punishment.

From the bedside, at least in my ER, men seem most prone to this last elision. Could be an observation bias, though, the deeper truth hidden behind what is easiest to see from where I stand. Often, though not exclusively, they are the ones brought in from fights, struggling to sit up in stretchers while hands try to hold their bleeding bodies down. They are the ones more likely to drink hand sanitizer, or the Chinese cooking wine sold at the small stores near my hospital, pass out on subway floors, then wake up in the minor hallway.

With time, they break social bonds, one at a time, with violence or lies, until their brother won't even answer the phone they're so alone, and they no longer have to worry about hurting anyone except themselves. The wounds they couldn't find a voice for are, finally, purely private.

I talked with an indigenous woman, an artist who took photographs of the reserves on which many native Canadians live. I lamented as we walked around her small show, the missing and murdered Aboriginal women in our country. We stopped at a series of billboards she had photographed, on which were plastered the names and likenesses of murdered men. Don't forget my brothers, she said to me, they are missing and dead in even greater numbers, and if you counted the ones lost to drink who are never coming home, you'd weep for them too.

Shortly after I graduated, I went to the funeral of one of my patients so determined to die that he visited the ER hundreds of times a year. As I was getting to know him, bearish, even dangerous when drunk, but when sober, smart and sweet, I gave him my one try.

"Doc. I started glue when I was ten. Been a drunk since twelve. I'm fifty now. It's who I am."

The next day, I heard his roar as the ambulance pushed him up the ramp. A few hours later, he walked back down the ramp and towards the corner store.

At his small funeral, I sat near the back, behind his family and friends, not sure how to explain why I was there. A sobbing sister took the lectern and explained the pain they had both endured at residential schools, the blessing that his was over. I left as she was done, and didn't speak to anyone. Since, others have taken his place and I've stopped going to their funerals. When I see them again, their breath sweet with mouthwash, stitches from another hospital left in a week too long, I look to make sure they've had no new trauma, take out the sutures, listen to their lungs, and write *discharge when steady*, though when they leave, they rarely are.

Sometimes I'll see the same patient twice in one day, even more, spitting, screaming, after a well-meaning pass-erby called an ambulance after thinking him, in a premoni-tion of his trajectory, dead. I wait until he sobers up enough to have a conversation about how he is killing himself, tell him it won't be long now. He stands, swaying at the thresh-old to the ER, slurring answers to my questions.

Occasionally, I can reach someone early enough in their life that they can remember what it was like before they made things worse by trying to feel better. Get some new friends, I say, as my best piece of advice, and they stagger from the ER, pushing off hallway walls.

It's a slow-motion tragedy, people rolling into minor hallway, vomit on their pants the first few years, then urine. We don't know how to help them. Theirs is an emergency for which we have lost the language if we ever knew it, but they come to this room all the same. Unless they say, right to our face, that they want to kill themselves that very minute, instead of just showing me they don't care if they live or die, we have little to offer except a list of detox centres and shelters. "They must *want* to get better," we tell ourselves, absolving our failure, ignoring that the precise problem, for many of them, is that they don't.

It's not just men who get lost in their hurt, or suffer it alone. A young woman, thirty, bruises and scars all over her back from falling against furniture. Her whole family, mom, dad, brother, were at her bedside, crying, telling me how they covered all the sharp edges with foam so she won't cut herself when she crashes, begged me to admit her. Her liver enzymes were sky-high already, even at her young age, but she shook her head no, no, I don't want to stay here. This isn't a prison, I said. Your place is. She left. Her mother put her face in her hands and wept.

Running away, or running towards. You might not even know.

I wrap a towel around my waist, go into the next room. On the floor, my red suitcase, clothes and cables and books scattered all around it. I sit in the pile.

I do a final shuffle of clothes, taking out a shirt or a pair of pants. I thread a string of safety pins, squeal off three feet of duct tape, fold it on itself, tuck these beside a folding knife. Headlamp. Battery. Carabiner. A loop of light climbing rope. I take the rope back out, toss it in the pile of discarded objects. This isn't MSF anymore. It's the city.

I toss in a padlock.

It's a bright winter day in Toronto, and sun beats through my window. I can hear car doors slam. I've more work to do today. After I run, I need to clear my apartment of all my books, all my clothes, move them into this room. I'm renting the apartment to strangers while I'm away.

"Don't let your lifestyle expand to accommodate your potential income," a teacher once told me, a final piece of advice before I left his emergency room to find a career of my own. "Then you get to be free."

I close my suitcase, satisfied.

K is for kind.

Women in bright scarves, glass beads glistening, struggle to fit overfull bags into the bins above. The sharpness of their perfume stings my throat.

The man in the row across from me is already sleeping, blanket pulled over his entire body like a shroud. The plane hasn't even taken off, and I can hear his soft snores. I hate him from four seats away.

A hand with small red nails reaches between the seats in front of me. Attached to it, the face of a young girl, hugging her mother's neck, eyes bright. I snap my jaws, as if to bite her finger. She giggles. Her mother pulls at her, and she disappears.

In the galley, flight attendants whisper in Amharic. The language has a lilting quality. It rises and falls, like a bird's song. It is a Semitic language, like Arabic and Hebrew, and it's hard for my mouth to get around the sounds. I know mostly travelling phrases. *Where is, how much. Left, right, straight, stop.* Numbers. *Thank you.* Amisehgenalo. Six syllables of gratitude.

What else? *Patient. Doctor. Hospital. Emergency. Fever. Pain. I'm sorry.* Suffering words.

A flight attendant laughs. A small hand creeps through the seats again, testing, hopeful.

The plane is nearly full. It is the only flight from Canada to sub-Saharan Africa, and families queue for hours, children at each arm while airline employees push towering boxes onto scales. Twelve hours in the air, and we arrive where it all began. Whatever journey humankind is on, it started in the Great Rift Valley.

Ethiopians are particularly proud of that. Lucy, *Australopithecus*, one of our oldest bipedal ancestors, sits in pieces in the basement of their national museum. She had spent most of the last decade in the U.S.A., the Ethiopians forced to be content with a plaster facsimile. No longer. She's back. This is the century where Africa recovers what has been lost to her. Bones. Doctors.

Ethiopia is claiming its role in this, as the only country in Africa that has never been colonized and, according to the Ethiopians, its most authentic voice. It is home to the African Union, has its own unique alphabet, cuisine, language. It is mentioned in the Bible, received the first Hijra of Muslims looking for safety, had its own population of wandering Jews, thousands of whom were airlifted to Israel in the early 1990s. In Ethiopia, these groups have shared space since you could claim such difference.

Even in the bustle of the city, there remain hushes of reverence carried from the past. In a traffic jam, horns all around, black smoke clouding your view, and a dozen women, wrapped in white, flit through on their way to church.

Addis Ababa, "New Flower," still deserves its name. It is barely more than a hundred years old. In that time, it has grown from a notion into a metropolis. Around five million people live inside borders that tumble wider every year. Like so many capitals, this one was founded on water, a set of hot springs a half day's ride from King Menelik's cool castle, swirling in clouds, high in the Entoto Mountains that rim the city. It has grown, though, these past decades, from a different kind of flow. Electricity, communications, people with money to put into banks and with planes to catch.

The historic centres across the country are more ancient, smaller, traditional intersections of different tribes and devotions. One of Ethiopia's spiritual homes, Lalibela, a wonder as grand as Machu Picchu or Angkor Wat, but even more remarkable, because it is still being used as it was when the first church was carved from solid stone.

Once, I followed a mountain path up to a stone church that wound its way along cliff faces so narrow in places that when I encountered a priest on his way down, I needed to retreat. He walked slowly forward as I reversed, his face lined by the harsh sun, staff in one hand. I found a wider place and stretched flat, my back against the cool rock. His robes brushed me. They smelled of frankincense and sweat. Below, the earth fell away, stretched to the horizon in black and green blocks that had been cultivated for millennia.

Eighty per cent of Ethiopians still live in the country-side, farming, watching the sky for rain. The urbaniza-tion that has drawn people into cities around the world, that is building Addis higher, has yet to reach many of them. It is on the way. What rooms will greet them should they fall sick?

Addis, in its short time, has developed into a lively intersection of people from all over the world. Ethiopia's land is older than history, though, and different tribes and peoples struggle to maintain identity within the bor-ders that now contain them. For the time being, despite this, and its sharing edges with a roll call of the world's most troubled states—Sudan, South Sudan, Somalia, Eritrea—things in Ethiopia are mostly peaceful.

Not at the margins, though. People are pinned by famine and by the wars that cause it. Once, if you needed to escape such places for more fertile ground, you could, let that place wither. Now, everywhere, land is claimed, and you're illegal, a refugee. Ethiopia hosts more of them than any other country in Africa, most of them from Sudan. Millions huddle just inside its bor-ders, clinging to safe space.

Its safest space, well, I'll be walking through it first thing tomorrow. Already the doctors in that tin ER are teaching each other lessons about how the young soldier, shot in the back, feeling so c-c-c-old, needs not blankets, but blood, no matter the side he claims.

The plane rumbles, shakes, lifts off. Toronto's grey pal-ette drops away. Ribbons of cars sift home. I shut the shade.

I watch a movie, write a few emails. I glance at my watch. Two p.m. in Toronto. Nine p.m. in Addis. Bedtime.

I fish at my feet, retrieve a black sack, zip it open. Inside is a plastic bag holding two sedatives with different onsets and durations, one quick but short, the other slow and long. I look to the man in the yellow blanket. He hasn't budged.

How the hell does he do that?

I order a glass of wine, drink the pills down, pull on my eye mask, and rest my head against the cool hull. It hums. Sounds stretch, then fade. The world closes in for good.

"Breakfast, sir?"

What? "Oh. Yeah. OK."

A smile, and a plate clatters down. In the crack between the seats, the girl in front clings to her mother, sleeping, head tilted back, carefree.

I lift the window shade. A meniscus of light is bleeding black from the sky. The Nile. Shadows of Sudan as dawn races into the morning.

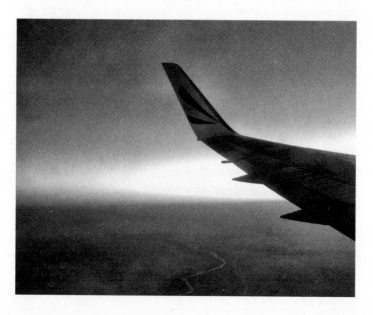

The light makes my eyes ache. As far as my body goes, this night will last all day.

I finish transferring all my contacts into a new phone. From "Ermias: taxi driver" to just: "Ermias." My friend.

I have made some there. It's the blessing I wanted to live when I agreed to return to the same place instead of a next troubled spot. Hands I get to touch again and again, the familiar faces of people I learn to know and love, who can see the challenges more cleanly than I would ever, meet them more deftly.

I've found it easier to be in Ethiopia than in other places where it's obvious I'm a stranger. In Sudan, or Dadaab, if I went to the market, people would notice. It's a strange feeling. I thought I blended. You'd never know you don't fit in unless someone points it out.

It's rare that anyone pays me special attention in Ethiopia, though, even in the countryside. One of my first times here, I asked someone about it, whether it was because of familiarity or pride. It's neither, he said. "We can tell by your skin that you are a rich man, but to us, you are just a man. Your actions show us who you are."

It seemed like a rule to live by.

The land racing away below is still full of anger and disease, people fighting about where they are from and the stories they were told. It is getting worse. Like my friends, I am watching war churn ever more violently through the north of Africa. Mali. Nigeria. Syria. Instead of tools, guns are being passed hand to hand.

The guns held in Libya, one of the largest caches in the world, disappeared from depots, re-emerged in souks, on Facebook for sale. Even big weapons are unaccounted for. Those with the least to lose are arming, then choosing a side. An epidemic of gunshots has followed, the wounded and hungry springing up quickly, as they do when human hands find triggers.

Although there is strain at Addis's expanding borders as buildings eat up land, the city's streets are safe. Few handguns, less booze, less cocaine—that's a main difference between there and Toronto. What makes a city safe is very much the same as what makes a person predictable.

In Addis, few people bother with weapons. Thus far, petty theft is about as bad as it gets. A taxi driver reached across to open my door, put his other hand in my pocket. A friend had a chain pulled from her neck. A couple of people I've taken to teach have "lost" their phones.

Once, working late in Black Lion, I went to the nearest restaurant and saw two young men, ferenjis, foreigners like myself. I struck up a conversation. They were visiting physiotherapy students, living on the sprawling Addis Ababa University health sciences campus that holds Black Lion and, recently, the country's only ER. They told me how one night, they were walking down the long, dark hill that leads from it, and a young boy grabbed the travel wallet from one of their open bags and darted down an alley. The boy was too fast to chase.

A taxi driver saw the exchange, pointed the young men to the same restaurant where I found them. A few minutes later, an old man, a neighbourhood patriarch, entered with a young translator, asked for a few details, and before their dinner came, returned with the wallet and flopped it down on the table, not a birr missing.

A street grift plays out near the hospital, with a group of boys. It is common for a son to be turned from his home at an early age, eight or nine, if a mother can't afford his mouth. A daughter helps with household chores, fetching water, and because she is more vulnerable to sexual abuse, is kept closer.

Some of the boys congregate in gangs to sort out together the business of living. At an intersection, near curio shops dangling with straw baskets and T-shirts, they lean on fences in ragged clothes, hair shorn into mohawks, plastic shoes two sizes too big or one too small, their feet as cracked and callused as an old man's.

The eldest, the ring's leader, hangs against a different fence, and with a whistle sends the youngest towards teams of Tilley-hatted sunburned ferenjis with black backpacks jutting in front of them. The boys approach with smiles that can't lose, holding a small box, a single pack of gum or tissues sliding back and forth in it. They hold the gum under the foreigners' noses, "Pleaseplease, mister . . . hungry," while underneath the cardboard blind, small hands fish through pockets.

It's not personal. It's a business. Pay attention, I tell the Toronto doctors who come to teach with me. Don't act like what you have doesn't matter, like you can afford to replace whatever you lose.

Before I fly, I do what I can to make sure Addis is the same as I left it last. I'm not with MSF this time, so I don't have the assurance of constantly updated security briefings. It is tough to know from the news. So far, the gathering wars have not played out in Addis. Each time I fly in, I look for signs that they are on the way.

The challenge for medical teams was once how to reach as many people as possible; now it's to neither be nor be seen as someone's proxy in a clandestine conquest, political or economic. The world's rich governments offer aid, and also weapons. With one hand they deliver vaccines, and with the other, create conditions for polio.

Since bin Laden was killed after he was identified by undercover operatives posing as part of a hepatitis B vaccination campaign, dozens of legitimate vaccine workers have been shot. Cases of polio, a disease nearly eradicated, surged in Pakistan. And now hospitals are being bombed. I can't remember that happening since I started to pay attention.

There are a few countries in Somalia right now, trying to hold the peace. Ethiopia is one. Al-Shabaab has promised them terror. Occasionally, on Twitter I learn about bomb threats on Bole road, Addis's main street, or an American friend will forward an email from the U.S. State Department warning Americans away from all shopping centres.

I don't go to malls. I don't stand at finish lines, or in crowds at football matches. The circles have started to close in for me too.

My ears feel full. The descent has started. I yawn. Crackcrackcrack. Below, terraced mountaintops, everything squared, not a corner left untouched. An occasional tree interrupts a line. Someone told me it is illegal to cut down living trees in Ethiopia, that only dead branches can be burned for wood.

A glimmer of glass and metal. The plane banks. Four separate stands of bright red-and-blue apartment blocks, a cloverleaf of roads connecting them. Neither were here last time I came. They are to make up for the homes that are coming down, the ones with mud walls and tin roofs that have been Addis since the beginning.

How much of a good thing can you take away and still know why it is there?

L is for love.

I'm walking to Black Lion. The morning sun is bright, but not yet hot. I pick my way along busted concrete piles, grey dust covers my shoes. Ahead of me, a woman in heels steps deftly from one boulder to another, black bag slung over her shoulder. Her eyes stay forward. She doesn't teeter.

Bole Road, Addis's largest artery, is broken. It's being torn up, crumbled, from the airport to Meskel Square, the wide open-air amphitheatre where holidays are celebrated, political speeches are made, and the best runners in the world start their mornings. Beside it, train stations are being pushed together, rows of old houses pulled apart. Cranes dangle on the city skyline in all directions.

Chinese engineers survey the progress, but it is Ethiopians who are driving the steamrollers. While the U.S.

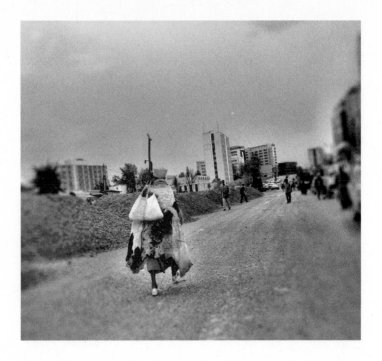

and Canada offer aid, China is helping with roads, railways. When last I left the city, children ran beside the open window of Ermias's car as it bumped down back roads, shouting, "China! China!"—a word synonymous with foreigner, and means.

I step onto flat ground and pick up my pace. I pass men with plastic-bag briefcases, women in groups of three, arm in arm. A goatherd threatens his animals with a switch, and they clamber over the median. A priest, his clothes made of hide, walks past, his head held high. No one looks at me. No one stares at their phones.

I look at mine. I'm going to be late. Shit.

At Meskel, I cross ten liquid lanes of traffic with five other people, each of us a few metres apart. If one steps, we all do. Cars squeal past in all directions, honking, narrowly avoiding us. My group of five spots a break and runs across the last few lanes, then falls out of step.

Along the sidewalk, men and women sell phone credits, loose cigarettes. There's a man with a display of electrical outlets on an orange tarpaulin, another with rows of sunglasses. I stop for a second.

At the base of the hospital hill, at the Churchill Road intersection, a half-dozen boys lean on fences. One of them, his hair in a high fade, its tips dyed blond, sees me, lets out a shrill whistle. A boy on the other side of the road looks to him, then me, reaches for the cardboard box beside him.

"Not even," I say, and shoo him back. The blond one smiles.

Up the hill, my breath comes fast. Salt beads on my lip. I pass banks. National police in woodland camouflage flank an official-looking building, guns held across their chests. A line of people sit on their haunches outside the Swedish embassy, papers in hand.

A high cement wall circles the campus. Near the hospital gate, a woman sweeps the sidewalk; behind her, a geodesic tarp home. A puppy, tethered to a wooden post beside it, wags his tail as I pass. The woman stops sweeping and smiles at me. I wave.

This family has been camped here the past couple of years. Each school day, about now, this woman sends her daughter off with a pink backpack full of books, school uniform fresh and clean. I must have just missed her. I'll start earlier.

A yellow bucket floats up from a street drain beside me, and her husband clambers out after it. He wets a rag in the rain water and starts washing a car. The driver leans in the shade of the hospital fence, toothpick in his mouth, waiting.

A dozen people are at the gate, pressing forward, pieces of paper in their hands. A man nearest the front is pleading with a guard I know. The guard hands a card back to the man, shakes his head, points at another entrance. He notices me, breaks into a grin.

"Doctor!" he says, grabs my hand, brings us shoulder to shoulder, in that way that Ethiopians have done since forever.

"Peace on you, peace on you. You're well? You're sure? Your family? They're well too? Everything's well? Are you sure? Good, good." The crowd waits. He claps me on the shoulder, drops the chain strung across the driveway, then raises it after I step over. Ferenji pass. Behind me, bargaining begins anew.

To my left, in a small courtyard, shaded by eucalyptus trees, nurses drink tea on broken white plastic chairs while sparrows brush the ground for crumbs and chatter in the branches. There's the old donated ambulance parked beside the ER, its tire still flat. I've never seen it move. A totem of good intentions fallen short of true action: a fully equipped ambulance given to a country with no medics to drive it.

In the ER's gravel parking lot, a blue Lada taxi lets off a limping man, a bloody cloth around his leg. He hops to a wooden bench. A family watches, crouched, elbows on knees, chins on hands, then turns their attention back to the body at their feet.

The ER: two tin rooms and a back hall. That's it, the place all this work is about, one that gathers people too sick for anywhere else. Dozens of times every day, cars from all over the country pull up to it, unannounced, with a dying person who has exhausted all their treatments. This place has a reputation as one where people go to die, rather than to get well. We see no sprained ankles, only badly broken ones.

At its entrance, another crowd, another guard. He is holding his arm across the threshold, looking away, entertaining no negotiations. I pass the side window, see bent heads around a triage desk, and keep walking. Although I'm curious to see what changes have crept into the room since I passed through it last, it is handover time. In a classroom a hundred metres away, the residents gather each morning to describe the night, tell stories of who lived and who died.

Students in white coats drift in and out of old concrete buildings. From one of them, a woman carries a large silver plate, emptied of the flat injera it once held. Some of the senior residents live there, two or more to a room. A few have electricity when it flows, even a hot plate. There is no running water.

My first time here, four years ago, I stood at the edge of the university grounds, halfway down this hill, with the dean of medicine. The hospital was behind us, grey, dark, teeming with people. Why can't you expand this way? I asked, gesturing towards the patchwork of brown tin roofs below us. Yes, he said thoughtfully, pretending he hadn't considered such an obvious prospect long ago. I talked with the minister for urban planning, the dean said, but was told there are too many people living there. How many? Three per square metre.

A bus pulls slowly by, and a man leans out the window, one hand on the steering wheel. "Hello, Dr. James!" he shouts, gives me a thumbs-up before shifting into second gear and pulling away.

I wave. When I first came, he was my driver, taking me from place to place in an old Land Cruiser. The assignment did not please him. It appears a promotion has had an effect on his mood. Or that I come back, tells him what kind of man I am.

I walk into a building five storeys high. On the glass that frames its foyer, exam marks are papered beside announcements, a request for a student to appear and explain her absence. The Office of Emergency Medicine occupies the basement. Life under the ground floor.

Kidist swirls clean water over concrete. I track through it, towards her. Her eyes fall to the ground, she stoops, smiles, says, "Hello, Dr. Jems," in a voice so soft I can barely hear it.

"Hi, Kiddy."

Down the dark steps, and I'm blind. I hear voices from the basement classroom. Halfway along a dim hallway is Dimile's small office, the department's secretary. It is black. No power today, no windows.

"Helloooo, Dr. J!" A silhouette rises from behind a cramped desk and gives me a gentle embrace. Even in the dark, Dimile's smile is wide and full.

I slide the door open, and it stutters in a familiar way. The track broke two years ago. There's no one to call for such things, no one who can remember who put that door in there, where they got it. The donors, more interested in opening day than opening doors, have moved on.

The intern at the front of the class stops mid-report. Facing her are fifteen residents in bright white coats, and in the front corner, Aklilu, the doctor tasked with making emergency medicine thrive in Ethiopia, and my oldest friend here. He is wearing, as always, a suit. He smiles, half rises, shakes my hand, whispers, "Good, good." I sit beside him.

The residents who know me smile too. The ones who don't study me for a second, then turn back to the young woman at the front of the room. She refuses.

"A twenty-five-year-old female from Oromia region presented with coma and abnormal body movement of one day duration after being struck by a lorry."

She stands and hands a thin black film to Aklilu. He nods, passes it to me. It's a CT scan of the head. There is blood spattered throughout it, signs of a swollen brain with no room to expand. When that happens, the brain pushes towards the only open space, the spinal canal in the ver-tebral column. The fine mesh of connections there, in the midbrain, get compressed, like the nerve in a leg held in one spot too long, except it is your breathing that falls asleep, your speech, the ebb and flow of your conscious-ness. If it does wake up, it's rarely perfect again.

The intern continues. Outside the high windows, a roar of traffic.

"We consulted the neurosurgical side, but they have no beds."

The hospital is always overfull, the equipment for some free operations must be donated, and its availability too sporadic to plan. People wait, sometimes for naught.

"What type of people get hit by cars?" I ask.

No answer. She waits. I wait.

"Most often . . . poor people," Yonathon says, finally. He has heard this question before.

"Sure. They spend more time there, don't they. You and I are at least sometimes driving, or on the bus."

They all agree.

"Did she need this scan?" I say, shaking it in my hand so it warbles. "It's expensive."

Yes. In case there was blood pushing in from the edges of her brain, pooling from a torn vessel. If that is the case, you see a white crescent, concave or convex depending on whether she's torn a pumping artery or a low-pressure vein. If you see either, a hole can be cut and the blood drained so the brain can reclaim its natural shape. If that's all there is, all the vectors of force caught by the skull, none cutting through the brain itself, then hallelujah, brother, happy day, your daughter may just love again.

"Does she need any more?"

No. There was no clot to remove, and even if there was someone to open up space for her brain to swell, an ICU to send her for a few weeks where a nurse could gently change the dressing over the fragile pink tissue until it shrank back down, there was no one to teach her to walk again even if she kept breathing.

"Will she live?"

Some of the interns, last-year medical students, look at each other. My senior residents shake their heads.

"No." I pass the black film behind me. A young woman holds it up to the bright window.

"Forty-five-year-old male presents with bleeding . . . Sixteen-year-old male with congestive heart failure . . .

Road traffic accident . . . The first death, a thirty-two-year-old man. Second death, sixty-four-year-old female . . ."

The intern at the front finishes the long list of sick-nesses. Aklilu and I interrupt a few more times, quizzing the ER residents, drawing out teaching points, then ask what supplies are missing, which patients need the most urgent attention.

We finish, and the intern sweeps her papers together. People start to stand. Aklilu motions them back down, introduces me.

"Thanks, Aklilu. Some of you know me. I'm here for the next few months. I will be in the ER to help most days, on weekends too. That's the good news. The bad news is, so will you."

In the first year or two, when I came to the ER un-announced, the triage desk would often be empty, and past it, a tired intern, still in medical school, surrounded by forty of the world's sickest, bleeding, seizing patients. After morning report, no matter how chilling, the resi-dents would retreat to the café on the hospital's main floor for tea and breakfast. I'm trying to pass on the urgency I feel in Toronto. There is still ground to claim. At night, the senior residents sometimes leave. Twenty-four hours in the dark ER, people tugging at your coat sleeve, is too much. In the darkest hours, an intern stanches bleeding until morning.

Attrition is high. Nurses, security guards, cleaners, all quit with great frequency. The ER is a place where they are sent as punishment, to think about what mis-takes they've made among the grieving. Students pass through, a tour of duty to the front lines, grateful to leave the dying behind when their month is up. At home, emergency medicine is one of the most competitive specialties for medical students, and most who apply won't get in. Here, no one knows why you would do it, because it appears that for the sickest, little can be done.

Aklilu sees ahead. This is his life more than mine, and it is him I am here to help. He knows there can be no transformation of a country without a place that cares for those hurt worst. All emergencies happen mostly among the poor. They are the ones crammed three per square metre trading rheumatic fever, the ones who tumble when the eucalyptus scaffolding buckles. Every year, after generations of trying, one billion climb above the poverty line. Every year, the same number fall below it. The most common reason for their drop? A health crisis.

Successes at addressing these crises in this tin room are rare, at least so far, but it is from it where the system must emerge. Until now, people with heart attacks died. Girls hit by lorries, too. Some in the hospital resent the stronger ER, because it is inconvenient. There are smart doctors at the bedside, feeling the urgency, calling at all hours. It has caused problems in friendships for some, their new role as advocate for people whose pain would once wait.

Three years of residents are in training now, fifteen total. My focus will be on the most senior group. I'll get them ready for the country's first exams, show them how to manage an ER, maybe even imagine a career. Should they last.

When the first five started, they spent long hours alone. No one had done what they were doing; they had no voice of experience to turn to for advice. Although we taught them the many ways they might save a sick person, the dying never stopped. Some of them started to miss shifts. One of them was gone for weeks with no warning. He came back a few times, then disappeared again. I tried to call him when I arrived this time, but the phone just rang and rang. There are four now.

It's different for the ones who started later. They knew someone who had faced their struggles, with a promise of more to join them. With camaraderie, an identity that buoyed spirits.

The residents come up one by one. "Yes, I'm good. My family too. I'm sure. Are you?" Smiles. We bump shoulders.

In the back, Biruk. He's one of the first four. His face is more serious than I remember, but still, the same soft eyes. He's bashful.

"Hi, Dr. James."

"Hey, my man. Good to see you."

"We're glad to have you back."

Behind him, Finot. Her smile takes up her whole face. She's newer, in second year, and one of the brightest. She understands what Aklilu knows, that to the family crouched on their knees, this place just up the road is more than a room. She is the first person you call if you can find no one else.

Biruk and Finot, in their mid-twenties, are the most experienced ER doctors in the country.

"Welcome, Dr. James," Finot says softly, leaning forward to touch shoulders. We all linger for a second, grinning at each other, not knowing what next to say.

"See you in there."

"Yes."

They leave. Aklilu and I talk for a minute, then follow. We pass Dimile, still sitting in the dark. "Welcome home," she whispers.

Up the short hill, even more full of students on their way to breakfast, past the concrete residences, to the gravel parking lot and the ambulance with the flat. The family with the body at their feet has gone or is inside. The man with the injured leg is seated on the plastic row of chairs, stick leaning across his lap.

The guard shouts, and the crowd parts. We move past. Most are family members of a patient already inside. We send families running to the labs that line the streets nearby, tubes of blood in their hand, or to load their injured daughter into a van owned by a company that sells CT scans to the sick. They return to this door, waving results through the open window, minutes or hours later.

A nurse stands, and from behind the triage desk, holds his forearm to me, so I don't need to touch his hands. I shake it. The sweet smell of sickness, bacteria and decay, carries past.

Patients lie on stretchers, some on the cement floor. Attendants crowd around their bodies. It is dim, even in the bright of day. Only a few windows to let in light, and the skylights are clouded with dust.

Behind a high counter, a group of young nursing students in white hats and coats stays the hell out of the way. No one is teaching them.

Ethiopia is intent on making the largest economic leap in the history of the world. They want to be a middle-income country by 2025. To this end, they intend to train ten thousand postgraduates in the next decade. In the previous one, they trained one hundred.

Of the thousands sent out of the country, to Europe or America, to get a PhD or to learn medicine well enough to teach it, just a small minority came back. A friend of mine studied medicine in Addis, and of his class of forty, only two practise in Ethiopia. Should the others return, their means and connections open doors in an increasingly international economy. Forget working in a hospital; they could now open their own.

The nation is tired of investing in students just to see them leave, so more universities are being built, medical school enrolment trebled. Students gather around patients three deep.

Aklilu is showing me the new monitor at triage.

"And these we made into resuscitation beds." He points to red-and-white-striped plastic curtains at the back, before pulling one aside.

The young girl struck by the lorry lies quietly. In her trachea, a plastic tube, a honeycomb of bloody bubbling in it. There are no ventilators in the ER, and the four in the intensive care unit, for the millions of people living three per square metre, are pushing breaths into others. The girl, at least for now, is breathing on her own, her tube connected to nothing.

Aklilu and I squeeze past the family, to her head. Her breaths come quickly, in bunches, then draw out into sighs. This pattern is a bad sign. The pressure in her brain is reaching its limit, pushing what keeps her breathing into a space too small to hold it. Her chest hitches.

A ribbon of gauze wrapped around her head, a bloody target at her temple. I pull down one of her lids. The pupils twitch. If seizures persist, large muscles tire, and the convulsion stops. Look to the eyes.

Biruk stands at the foot of the bed. He spent last night here.

I direct him to the head, show him the saccades of her irises.

"She kept on with her seizures all night," he tells me, "so we gave her some Valium, but didn't want her to stop breathing."

I ask Aklilu and Biruk about different intravenous medicines, ones that work on seizures, and they shake their heads. They know what I'm talking about, but to now there have been too few people asking for it for any of the pharmacies to stock it. There is one that comes in pills, Biruk says. We decide to crush some, put them into her stomach with a tube, but we all know she is dying.

The family looks at us, wide-eyed. An older woman, an aunt, a mother, wipes the snot dripping from the girl's nose with her skirt. An older man wearing plastic sandals, one red, one blue, his feet callused at the buckles, holds her hand.

"Do they understand?" I ask Biruk. He nods.

He has aged. The boy I met is long gone. Sorry, brother.

Biruk says some words in Amharic.

Tears well in the father's eyes. We move on.

Residents in white coats lean over patients, listening for trouble in hearts and lungs. No computers. Aklilu leaves to attend a meeting, and Biruk folds his coat under his arm, ready to return to his bed for some sleep. I stop him.

"You did good, man. It was the right thing to do to intubate that lady. I would have done the same thing."

He smiles softly, and walks past the growing crowd of patients at the metal door waving their hospital cards.

M is for middle.

Patpatpat. Rain on a metal roof above me. My body feels impossibly heavy.

Bed. Curtains. Street light.

I close my eyes again.

Wait.

Where the fuck am I.

A thin bright thread of awareness slivers between me and dreamless sleep.

Wake up.

I shake my head, open my eyes wide, prop myself up on my elbow. Details grow clear. Suitcase. Pile of books.

Addis. It's night. Broke my travel rules, slept the day through. Felt so good. There are few experiences as exquisite as a jet-lagged nap. Gets you right where you want to go, no foreplay, just deep subconscious.

I lie on my back again, listen to the din above me. It rises and falls in waves. When it slows, music carries through the wall from the room next to mine. Piano, a woman's muffled voice, then the rain, patpatpat.

I've been here a few days, but it feels longer. There are few pulls from home. It's true that though there are differences here, there are many familiarities. Taxicabs, sparking neon signs.

Emergency departments. Gave Aklilu a day off from it today. He normally comes in on weekends, sorts shortages of EKG paper, brokers arguments between consultants, and helps with the sickest.

I filled in for him as best as I could. Demelesh was the senior resident working, seeing which of the dozens of people stuck in the ER for days might be well enough to go home, then the new cases dropped off in the parking lot.

As of yet, there's not much flow in the ER, nor through it. Demelesh draws most of the blood, infuses the drugs families have trotted back from the pharmacy. During the week, there are more people to help, but it has yet to assume the twenty-four-hour integrity of a human body, functioning at full capacity regardless of the hour. Worse, if a person in a diabetic coma comes in, once he gives her fluid and insulin, he cannot hand the rest of her care over to a consultant so he is freed to concentrate on a feverish man. Instead, he cares for both, sometimes for days. We've yet to convince enough people in the hospital that the greatest prize the world can claim is an empty emergency bed.

It's not a problem unique to Addis. Crowds surge to cover every square inch of public emergency rooms, no matter where they are. LA. Khartoum. A difference is that, over time, the ER is known as a bellwether for how each part of the system shoulders the shared work of moving people through, and if it gets stuck, everyone must move.

Such growth is something to believe in, sure, but it requires investment bigger than any one person, even fifteen who know just what do. You need ambulances and oxygen, enough to cope with a surge, waiting ICU beds, people who check the expiry date on drugs, stock those boxes of tubes the size of your little finger, consultants committed to taking patients out of the ER even if it means hosting them in their hall. Without these, it never becomes much more than a room.

This morning, in its many waiting faces, I saw a woman, from the countryside, tattoos of devotion on her face and neck. She was breathing up and down as if she was running a race.

Demelesh and I had talked to many people before we reached the foot of her bed, and I was only half-paying attention, drifting in and out of the dreams, until Demelesh turned from Amharic to English.

"Doctor James?"

"Hmm?"

I looked up. She stared at me. The dreams fell away. I recognized her.

And she knew me, though we had never met. I can't explain it. There was a deep familiarity I had only known a couple of times in my life. We were looking at ourselves.

She was too breathless to lie down, because the tops of her lungs were the only place water wasn't. Rheumatic heart disease. Her heart danced fast on the one monitor that worked, and her hands were pale and cold from the dopamine, an adrenalin-like drug Demelesh was dripping into her a bit at a time to squeeze her vessels tight, get blood to her brain. She was tugging at her oxygen mask, her eyes locked to mine, pulling it away, a late sign as serious as saying she was so cold. Her face, though, held no fear, only determination. She turned away, finally, burrowed her forehead into her father's neck.

There were no ventilators. We had seen two people already who needed one, and we were only half through the crowd. The girl hit by that lorry, her breath even weaker than the other day, a man who was slowly being paralyzed from the feet up. Soon, in a day or a week, his diaphragm would stutter and he would be breathless.

The woman's father was a farmer, and a private hospital was well beyond his means. He had likely spent what money he had travelling here, and was losing even more of his daily bread with each passing hour. We peered through her back with an ultrasound, saw lakes of fluid pressing her lung, so Demelesh pierced her back with a needle, took off five syringes of cloudy water. It didn't help. Every time we came back to the bed, her blinks lasted longer and even with the dopamine, her blood pressure became too low to measure. She leaned harder into her dad.

We talked about intubating her, giving her father the bag to squeeze. It never works, Demelesh said. I know, I answered. Plus, she has HIV, Dr. James, and it looks like TB and rheumatic heart disease, so even if she lives today,

she will die soon. I know, I said again. He suggested we
palliate her, keep her comfortable. OK, Demelesh. We
moved away.

We saw the rest of the people, no one near as sick,
made plans for the rest of the patients. I stopped by her bed
again. She was pressed to her father's chest. Her fingers
were white at the tips. I told Demelesh to call me if she got
any worse, though there wasn't much room for that. I
didn't know what I would suggest, I just wanted to know.

I turn over in bed, and check my phone. No missed
calls. No messages

Was she twenty? Maybe. Hard to tell. She was so
thin. Chronic disease will eat you until there's almost
nothing left.

You'll read that life expectancy in Ethiopia is in the
sixties. That doesn't tell you the true story, because it's
not a constant attrition, year by year, with most dropping
surrounded by grandchildren. It's an average. It's those
who die young, as children, or in delivering them, who
pull it down. If you could have saved them, just that one
time, the chances are you would change their fate completely and they would live a long life.

I open the door to my small balcony. No music, just
the trickle of water pouring down the eaves. Below me,
a newly paved section of Bole, slick with rain, asphalt
still bevelled.

The construction is moving so fast. The road will be
thick with traffic in no time.

Fat drops slash past street lamps, bounce off the
black ground. A man dashes from one awning to the next,
a piece of cardboard held over his head, then disappears

between a break in a corrugated wall. The street is empty again. I shiver, shut the door, turn back to bed.

I look at my phone again.

Fuck it. I'll pay for her.

I pick it up, dial Demelesh.

I never do this. It's not realistic to make it a practice. The point is to be present for the difficulties the residents face as truly as possible, not buy a way around them. I don't bring supplies, or give out dollars. I tell myself it skews local economies, bypasses innovation, sets expectations. Or maybe I just say that because it allows me to say no.

"Demelesh. Hey, it's Dr. James. Look, I figured . . . that woman with the tattoos, if her father can't afford a private ICU bed, I can . . . You did? She is? . . . Wow, that's great news. Good work. OK, call me whenever you want. Bye."

Huh. He went to the ICU and argued her into a bed. Maybe he saw something of himself in her too.

I'm elated. I stand up, then I sit down, then stand up again, open the balcony door, shut it. I can't stay still.

The rain has slowed. The music through the wall has changed to Ethiopian jazz. I pry the cap off a bottle of beer, St. George, and take a long drink. A buzz blossoms in my heart, my face, thousands of tiny bubbles.

N is for nutrient.

I'm blinking blearily in morning report, straining to hear Finot's soft voice. Aklilu was called out of the room to attend urgent business. His is work for six in Toronto. Few people who have means to leave linger in the public system, let alone the country. Should they, their jobs are many. He gave me a soft promise to take a vacation during my months here.

"Maybe a few days," he said. "To visit my family."

Finot's voice: ". . . Three patients kept in the ER. A twenty-four-year-old male who presented with a three-day history of bleeding from his nose . . ."

I saw this man yesterday, when I came back from lunch. He was sitting quietly, in a corner, easy to miss. He sat where my grandfather would be, at the edge, waiting, watching, not wanting to intrude. He had the clothes one sees in the countryside, and the same silence.

He leaned forward on a stool, eyes closed, one hand pinching his nose, the other holding a shepherd's stick. The front of his cloth tunic was black with dried blood.

Simeh manuh? *What's your name?* Ahmed, he whispered.

". . . his heart rate at presentation was 130. He was shivering . . ."

Aklilu skitters the classroom door open, sits back beside me.

". . . we started an intravenous and gave him one bag of fluid, and his heart rate slowed . . ."

The man was a goatherd from a day away. He brought with him no one who could donate blood or run across the street to pay for tests. He had no money to offer. A friend of his, a health officer in the only clinic miles from his home, gave him the address of this place, maybe just the name of the hospital, Black Lion in Addis Ababa.

He had a few birr, enough for the bus, promised a goat if his friend watched his flock. Minivan to minivan, people shrinking from the growing stain on his front until he sat on the ground outside the tin room.

No one bargained with the guard on his behalf, so he waited hours until a nurse noticed, and beckoned him forward. He stood, shaky, dizzy, almost fell, caught himself with his stick, and walked to her.

The guard shooed people aside until Ahmed could sit on the triage stool, and the nurse put her hands on his wrist, felt his heart faintly thrumming with small fast pulses.

We took two of the last units from the blood bank.

"... before transfusion his hemoglobin was 30 ..."

As low as I've seen. My hemoglobin was 140 last time I checked. When it gets too low, even though there might be water enough to push around, there are too few cells to hold oxygen tightly, so they must do double duty, move even faster.

"... white blood cell count, 3. Platelets, 5 ..."

Everything's low. It's his bones. Their marrow has stopped pushing out cells, all of them. It's the lack of platelets that is making his blood so thin.

"... there were no platelets in the hospital. His colour improved with transfusion, and he felt better ..."

Great. Now we need to find—

"... about three hours ago, though, he started to vomit blood ..."

Ah fuck. I massage my temple with my fingers.

"... his heart rate is again almost 120. We were unable to find more blood at this time and he remains in the ER."

Finot stops, looks at me and Aklilu.

Aklilu turns to the rows of white-coated young doctors. The ones at the back, unable to hear a word, are staring at the ceiling. Their heads swivel to attention. The ER residents are at the front, silent, listening, waiting.

"Gelaw?"

"Well, he now has gastric bleeding, and is in shock ... He needs blood, platelets, and possibly ... an endoscopy?"

A camera, to look in his stomach, to see if there is bleeding that can be stopped, an ulcer cauterized. It is a good answer, but from a book written in the future.

"True," Aklilu says. "All of those things would be good. But there's none we can do now."

Eyes are all forward now.

"Where is the blood from?" Aklilu asks.

Whispers from the back.

"Thrombocytopenia." Low platelets. "Coagulopathy." Thin blood, liver failure. "Varices." Vessels swollen and weak from trying to feed a scarred liver, burst in the esophagus.

"Possible," Aklilu says. "Not the type to have liver problems, though."

Occam's razor. One should not multiply possibilities unnecessarily. The many ways a sickness shows itself are most often due to a single disease rather than two or more. With "never say never, never say always," a balance of medical heuristics.

"Gastritis." An inflamed stomach, the tissue raw and swollen. "Mallory-Weiss." A tear in the mucous membrane of the esophagus from retching.

The students are proceeding stepwise, approaching sicknesses anatomically. Blood problems, liver, one's stomach, throat. It is one of a few ways to structure knowledge in medicine. Another is to categorize varieties of insults, *how* weak spots wear through, rather than in which places. Trauma, infection, cancer, nutritional. Lists don't work. Our brain flows best in branches, splitting and splitting, like the neurons that make it.

"Could be. But what can we do today?"

"Endoscopy," two people say at once.

The senior ER residents shake their heads. There's no

one to do it, maybe only a few in the country who could, none of them used to patients this sick. Not yet.

"No. What else could it be?"

The teaching in medicine is often Socratic. You are taught to ask deeper and deeper questions, to constantly challenge every assumption. What emerges is not the answer, necessarily, but more questions on the endless path of trying to do right for the person in front of you.

Aklilu looks at his watch. He is getting frustrated. "What was his presentation?"

"Bleeding," Biruk says.

"From where?"

"His nose. He could be vomiting the blood he has swallowed."

"Yes."

His stomach is full of his own blood, chewing it up. The iron is an irritant. We can't be sure, but I hope so.

Biruk continues. "So we stop the blood from his nose. With pressure. Pack it with gauze, give him some antinauseant."

It is a good emergency plan. Even if you aren't sure what's wrong, you do what you can. It's very common, even at home, to manage without a diagnosis. Plug what's leaking, worry about the cause later.

I try not to opine about home much. Not only would it detract from the good work done here, but what we do at home isn't always good medicine. We would arrange for an endoscopy without marrying likelihoods and expense. And if we did, it would be as an esoteric exercise, pushing any hard decisions as far into the future as possible.

On my last shift at St. Mike's, an old woman was struck crossing the road. Her head was full of blood. Her blood pressure dropped while she was in the CT scanner, and as I watched the x-rays slice through her pelvis, a blush of contrast bloomed on the screen from a jagged break in her groin.

She was bleeding to death too. In the ICU, they gave her unit after unit of blood, twenty in total, called in a radiologist and a team of people, put a catheter into her leg, found the bleeding vessel, and stopped it with a foam plug. She died six hours later from her head injury, with good blood pressure.

You are able to do that at home, because you don't see the dollars. Here it is clear where each one comes from, because it is pulled creased and tattered from some worried mother's pocket. It makes the math of what a life is worth very clear: everything to those who love you. Once you see through the lie that the worth of a person's life depends on where they were born, or how close to money, you never go back to being the same person.

"If the man was an alcoholic, would you think differently?"

Nods. We discuss liver failure, how it swells the vessels, causes a different type of bleeding. The treatment would be different then. Vitamins, plasma rich with clotting factors from another person's arm dripped into his.

We plan to stuff this man's nose tight with gauze, give him some fluid until we find more blood, and hope his heart can slow down, at least a bit. It's tough to watch a young man bleed to death, but without saying so, we plan for that too.

Aklilu excuses himself. Finot continues with the list of patients she saw, an inventory of broken men and women, then passes around their pictures. We hold black films high towards the basement windows, look for smooth white lines that no longer connect.

The last one is passed around. I thank her for her hard work. We all stand.

"I'll see you in the ER in a few minutes," I tell them.

They leave the room and crowd the small hall, murmuring to each other, some smiling, arm in arm, a tide of white coats. It's easier here during the day. Nights alone are long.

I pass Dimile's windowless office. She turns her phone light on so I can see her face.

"No power again today?" I ask, rhetorically.

She shakes her head, makes a pouting face.

I climb the stairs and head towards the main hospital. In its foyer is a buzzing coffee shop where I like to wait as the residents talk to their patients in Amharic before passing on to me what they learned.

I sit on a torn red stool, signal for an espresso. In addition to the oldest bipedal primate, Ethiopia lays claim to coffee too. Only a few million years after Lucy made her final walk, a goatherd noticed the liveliness of his animals after they ate certain green beans, tried some for himself, and he herded harder then he'd ever herded before. Centuries later, in the 1940s, Mussolini tried to make a home here. The Ethiopians beat him back, but kept the espresso machines.

I sip one slowly. A pair of students in short white coats ask if they can share my table. I nod. They start speaking excitedly in Amharic. The waitress interrupts, listens to their order. They stand, walk to an outside sink to wash their hands.

It is an act that borders on ritual here. People who have never travelled to places like Ethiopia or Sudan have misconceptions that they are dirty, that the people know no better. The opposite is true: people are more careful because there is not yet a system to allow them to be careless. It is the risk that is much higher.

In the modern world of philanthropy and assistance, it is much easier to get international money for specific sicknesses, because successes are easier to measure, numbers simpler to manipulate. One of the reasons Black Lion has monitors, those striped curtains, the learning centre, is that the American government helped Addis Ababa University prove that a high proportion of people with HIV sought care at Black Lion. Having water to wash your hands, or platelets for goatherds who are bleeding to death, requires a different calculus.

My tablemates have returned. I smile, drain the last grains of sugar from my cup, and gesture for the bill. I pull four torn single-birr notes from my pocket and place them on the table, 20 cents, and the waitress adds them to a thick stack in her apron's pouch. Beside me, my two table-mates tear off a piece of injera, expertly fold it between their fingers, and start pinching up bites of chickpea stew.

It is a fasting day in Ethiopia. For Orthodox adherents, about half the population, this means one meal on these days, containing no animal products. It happens twice each week, and during Lent's fifty-five days. Many Ethiopians are vegan for at least a few months of the year, have been so for millennia. With the Muslim population fasting for Ramadan, asceticism is part of everyone's life, its intention to keep a person alive to indulgences, to low-level chronic addictions to food, sex, intoxicants, entertainment.

Few Ethiopians I've met fast from injera, or at least not for long. It is eaten at every meal, is both plate and utensil. It is made from teff grass, its seeds as small as a poppy's. It takes many hours of labour to thresh the grass, separate the seeds from the stalk, winnow them, then pound them into dust. The flour is fermented into a batter, which is then poured onto a hot skillet, making a giant pancake that forms the staple diet for nearly all Ethiopians and Eritreans. It is high in calcium, iron, protein, free from gluten. Nutritional anthropologists suggest that it is the grass, and the injera from it, that has allowed the Ethiopians to flourish in a place where vitamins otherwise are scarce.

Last I heard, both teff grain and flour are banned from export. Ethiopia wants it all. It is legal to export injera, though, and twice a week, hundreds of rolls are unloaded in Toronto. Those of us with a taste for it know what days these flights arrive.

The most common question asked when returning from months away, after the impossible "How was it?" is "What did you eat?" In Ethiopia, injera. There is no choice. You must love it. Luckily, I do. In Sudan, it was beans and potatoes, a combination less prone to enthusiasms. In Kenya, Dadaab was too dry for any other animal save camel, so we ate those. Even in the hottest months, they plodded towards us past cattle bones that littered the sand like white shipwrecks and we stewed their tough flesh, dry from all the miles.

Our cook there told me that before you kill a camel, you must ask its permission. If it agrees, it lowers its neck and cries a tear. If it refuses, it raises its head away from the blade, and you release the tether. On the other side of the barbed wire wall, people ate sorghum, or nothing at all.

My first thought on return to Toronto is also of food: so much. Bakery next to convenience store next to restaurant next to coffee shop. Having solved with such dramatic effect the problem of food scarcity, we've created another: perpetual craving.

We have too much of everything. A friend of mine cuts out parts of people's stomachs, because they can't stop overeating. He says by the time these patients leave hospital, they are off most of their medicines. At St. Mike's, overdoses—food, alcohol, drugs—are much more common than deficiencies. Still, well people grind smoothies with vitamins and microchemicals, hoping to fill some newly discovered nutritional crevice and reach a new peak.

It is likely the bleeding man has bone marrow failure from a deficiency of some kind. A friend of mine, Gena, a hematologist here in Ethiopia, told me that she sees people like him all the time. With no corner shops or cooling freezers, people must eat what grows around them, and since most people these days grow single crops for money, if little else grows, or the sun stays hidden a week longer than usual, there is little variety. With a simple vitamin, she tells me, the cells recover after a few months.

You can almost forget how vulnerable a life is if not given the conditions to thrive. Once, a boy I knew was strapped to his mother's back on a long, treacherous walk from war. He maintained a steady diet of nothing for weeks. His skin fell off. We gave his mother soft blankets, because every time we turned him it would slide off his back like tissue paper on a wet windshield and stick to the bed, dry, then flutter away. Underneath, his body was white. Every single thing was falling away. He would neither eat nor cry. We poured rich milk through his nose, into his stomach, and it wouldn't even catch, would just come out the other end twenty minutes later, undisturbed.

I looked for answers to his problem, one I had never seen before, that my professors in school had not imagined. I read textbooks and searched scholarly articles on "total body desquamation" or "generalized epithelial sloughing AND malnutrition." The closest I could find was a case study where a gastroenterologist packed his camera on a plane and took endoscopic bites from the intestines of starving children. The cells that pulled food in, pressed flat on a glass slide, looked pale, weak, and faded under the microscope. They had a similar anemic appearance to chronic inflammation. Everything was withered. Skin on the outside, skin on the inside.

One morning, I came to work, and his family had taken him home to die. I left shortly after, landed in Geneva, walked to the MSF office past stores selling algae and alkaline water, sat waiting with four others to talk about the things we had seen to some of the few people who understood.

I walk slowly up the gentle hill towards the ER, squeeze past the crowd of patients being ignored by the guard. I see my team gathered around the young, bleeding man. His eyes are white. He shivers in the corner. Fresh blood is on his tunic.

No platelets. He'll need more red cells. We send someone to start the long process of finding what we can, begging, borrowing, and move on to the next bed.

O.

It's a type of blood. Universal donor. It has neither A- nor B-type proteins on the surface of its cells, and therefore avoids being recognized by a new body as once belonging to someone else.

We need some.

I'm standing next to the bed of that bleeding man watching the last of what we have drip.

Drop. Drop. Drop.

A line of red cells tumbles towards Ahmed who, even with his black skin, is as pale as a ghost. That's where the saying comes from, I'm sure. Not some gauzy spectre at the top of the stairs, but the bleached lips of the newly dead.

Drop. drop. dr . . . op.

A drip dangles. I roll the tube between my fingers. The blood hangs. You must watch it all the time. I learned to do this in Sudan, where the wind was so hot, blood would clot in the tube before it could drain into a person's arm. I take a syringe, fill it with some sterile saline, and flush the IV. It starts to flow slowly again. A nurse nods.

With me is a young doctor, an American, in Addis for a month to learn how to do this type of medicine, where minutes matter and you've none of the stuff. She arrived unannounced, and unsupervised. I saw her, one afternoon, peering over people's shoulders, trying to fit in.

"How the hell do you know when to leave?" she mutters under her breath, looks at all the patients around us, her watch, and joins me in watching the drops.

Biruk is at the head of the bleeding man's bed, untangling a mask. Clear wires run around his hand as he tries to trace them to the scuffed metal canisters that sit in a row, like round memorials, behind patients' beds. He listens to one for a hiss, drops it, listens to another.

The man is breathing quickly. His heart rate is almost 150. Finot told me that he had started shitting blood too. Maybe it wasn't from his nose after all.

There are still no platelets.

"How you doing up there, Biruk?"

"Can you tell me the saturation?" he says, sweating, trying to crane his neck to see the numbers on the one working monitor, a few beds away, where we have stretched the cable over to the young man's finger.

"Not reading," I say.

"How's the IV coming, Finot?"

"It's OK," she says, bent to the man's elbow, and slides the plastic cannula over the needle. A nurse hands her some clear IV tubing, and she screws it on.

"Does he have a pulse in that wrist?" Biruk asks.

"One minute," she says, taping the IV in place. She feels along the underside of his wrist, groping, pauses, shakes her head. "Feeble."

Blood pressure is low. He's lost much more blood than we've been able to give him. The unit I was watching is almost finished. The hospital is hungry for it today. Finot visited both the OR and the blood bank again this afternoon, to beg for this one. What is left is for the operating theatre. The system is still stretching to accommodate people off the street surviving long enough to need more.

"Femoral pulse?"

She presses a gloved hand hard into the man's pelvis. She nods.

The arteries are bigger there than in the wrist, a low blood pressure easier to feel. If he had had no pulse there, she would have tried to feel the one in his neck. If no beat there, the heart is too empty to push a pulse even a few centimetres.

The man trembles as he takes in a sighing breath. Biruk spins a flow valve onto a new oxygen tank. A huff of air bursts as the seal breaks. He pulls a used mask over Ahmed's face, two round rolls of gauze stuck into his nose.

A: okay for now.

B: not great.

C: fucked.

More salt water in his veins to keep the pulse full, though it has none of the richness that he needs.

D, a drug to lessen his bleeding stomach's acidity, in case it is dissolving the clot. The evidence isn't that great for it. Well, actually there's none, but it's unlikely to hurt. A nurse leaves to search the pharmacy.

When I first travelled this floor, five years earlier, Aklilu by my side, the cupboards were nearly bare of drugs, and the defibrillator, the machine that shocks a stopped heart, was broken. There was no suction machine, nor anyone to know when to use it.

"This will all change," Aklilu promised, and somehow, it has. Another university brought monitors, training materials, equipment. The Ministry of Education committed students, the Ministry of Health, supplies. We brought teachers. Aklilu persuaded five students to join a specialty no one had heard of to work on a problem no one knew was there. A dozen nurses are enrolled in an emergency master's, one of them sitting at the front today, taking blood pressures, asking questions.

Slowly, a frame is emerging. Last week, a young man came in the front doors, lips as pale as Ahmed's, a dab of blood on his chest where a screwdriver had pierced his heart. Finot did an ultrasound, saw the slick of blood pooling in the fibrous pericardium, from a hole in the heart, collapses, causing it to short of a full beat.

She and I put masks over our faces and went up two floors to the OR and walked in on a surprised surgeon putting in last stitches. She tied her knots quickly and cleaned the table for this boy, cut his chest open, closed the wound. The hole, though, was through a heart vessel, and as it was cinched, his heart fibrillated, and he died. Closer, ever closer.

Ahmed trembles below me, oxygen whistling over his face. Biruk places a piece of white tape on the mask's edge, to keep it from sliding off.

Up to this point, the ER has been given no particular priority, despite the precariousness of the patients we see in it. Last week, I went to the small repair office in the basement to see how much more time was needed to fix the EKG machine, and found two men mending an office chair.

I never thought I would be like this, studying different ways to triage repair requests. I thought I would just do medicine in the bush, triaging people, writing about them if there was time. Somehow, it's about systems now. Just as there are veins to bring blood back to the heart, there is one for ambulances that shuttle the injured towards repair. This is why many aid efforts fall short: they perpetuate hierarchy. Instead of creating conditions for natural growth, they add pieces at the top, from somewhere else, and blame the environment when they don't fully connect. Life doesn't follow straight lines. It emerges.

The drops have stopped. The bag of blood is done, only a smear left in it. The man's heart rate has fallen to 120. What hints of panic there were in his face have retreated.

Finot, the American, and I sit at the desk, talking about the category of shock the man is in given his response, how many litres of blood he has likely lost, how many he is still missing. The estimate, I tell them, comes from experiments done on greyhounds that were cut open and left to bleed to death, did you know that? They shake their heads. During the First World War, doctors used to bleed patients like this one. Can you believe that? They couldn't.

"No answer," Biruk says, hanging up his phone. He has been trying a number for one of six people in the country who might put a camera down into this man's stomach and determine if there's bleeding to be stopped.

Around the corner comes a resident, a wide smile on his face. In one hand, a bag of bright red blood. In the other, an even greater prize: a straw-coloured bag of platelets.

"I found them in the hematology clinic. A patient didn't show for his transfusion," he says, proudly offering them both to Biruk, who beams, comes around from behind the bed, takes the bags, sets them down, and gives the young doctor a hug.

"See, Dr. James," he says, still holding the young man's hand. "This is a great guy."

I agree, and the two of them hang the bag, start dropping the cells back in.

P is for practice.

Pulled the muslin gauze over the face of a thirteen-year-old girl and walked down the hospital's dark halls, up four flights of stairs to find some light.

In a doorway, a woman with bright sequins on her hijab smiled at me, a beautiful baby on her hip. Framed by a window, two lovers held hands, looking at the city that stretched below. I put one of my hands on the wide sill. It was warm with sun.

Write hard and clear about what hurts. That's what Hemingway said, anyway. Sunsets, murmurations, those friends, walking hand in hand, five floors below, already broken. The panicked eyes of a girl over an oxygen mask twice too big.

Frantic is a better word. She was clawing at her mother.

First the fear, then the fade. Remember? Contagious as ever, that feeling. It makes me want to, even now, put my fist through this window in front of me, just to let the cool air in where it belongs.

Do you have enough money to visit a private intensive care unit? one of the young doctors asked. Ours are full.

You already know this part of the story. The family stepped away to count their money.

Her kidneys had failed, and now her breathing was too. I looked at the monitor. Her heart's electricity was wide and irregular. It would soon disappear.

We had given her what we had at hand. It wasn't working. I turned back to her. Her eyes were closing.

She can't breathe like this much longer.

I'll get the airway box.

We get the box when we can't bear to watch another person die right then, we use it to practise for better days.

I put my hand on the girl's sharp shoulder. It's OK, I said. You'll be OK.

She heaved in my hand, then turned to me. I'm too tired, you take over, she said, stopped breathing, and vomited a gallon of water.

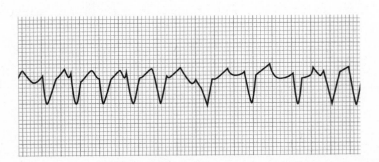

I laid her down, turned her small face to the side, let it pour out and onto my shoes. Her head fit perfectly into my hand. I touched her neck. She had a pulse

Dawit, come here. Take her head. See? Right there. Don't lean the blade on her teeth. No no. You're leaning. You'll break them. Pull up, towards the corner of the room. Good.

He passed the tube into her trachea. Her heart stopped.

You, I pointed at a nursing student, start CPR.

Faster.

Deeper.

Stand on a chair.

The bed was too soft for us to squeeze her heart. A nurse came running with a cupboard door and slid it under her, so we could crush her heart against the wood.

Adrenalin, please.

The electricity came back, disappeared. The IV jerked out of the vein from all of the rocking, and a small balloon of water appeared in her wrist. I jutted a needle deep in her groin as she bounced up and down, searching for a vessel I couldn't see. I hit bone. It's an unforgettable feeling, a smooth scraping, all wrong. I withdrew, stabbed again, pulled hard on the syringe, but no bloom of blood. I looked to her feet.

They were a little girl's. You could tell because her toenails were painted red. The colour was cracked, faded, only patches here and there.

It's the little things that hurt, because they are windows into something much, much bigger.

Someone found a vein in her wrist.

Sodium bicarbonate, please.

Pulse? Wait. Yeah, I can feel it. It's back. OK. Stop CPR. It's gone. Start. Stop. Start.

It just wouldn't stay. We spent an hour on that cupboard door, switching back and forth, straddling her chest, using Adrenalin and atropine, and no one wanted to quit, even after her eyes widened into the stare of the dead, and the flesh behind her red toenails blanched white.

Stop CPR.

We stepped from behind the curtain, found the family gathered in a tight circle in the hallway. Dawit told them. Thank you, her uncle said, in English, tears in his eyes. A family of cousins nodded, yes, yes, thank you. I nodded back, confused.

For what?

A nurse took the door from beneath the girl's body and around the corner.

Dawit and I sat in the small, cramped office in the back of the ER hallway with the nurses and the medical student who'd helped with CPR. We talked about what happened, how we might do better next time.

It would be good if the airway equipment was nearer.

Yeah. Suction too. It took too long.

A central line instead of those small IVs.

Blood work.

Ultrasound.

Ventilator.

Dialysis.

We fell quiet. Outside the door, the murmur of the ER.

Did you see the paint on her toenails? someone asked.

Yes, everyone whispered, yes.

Let's plan to do a practice resuscitation in a day or two.

Sure, sure.

We all stood up. The nurses filed out.

Dawit, I called out.

Yes, Dr. James.

It's important to be sad, I said. He nodded, walked back into the ER.

We spend the day busy with other things. Another woman, from days away, came in vibrating with each throb of her overlarge heart. We slowed it down, and her pressure returned to her wrist. A man bitten by a dog a month earlier, brought in by his wife, gagged when we offered a bottle of water. Hydrophobia. Rabies. Fatal. He left when our backs were turned. A woman sagged in a chair. She noticed me noticing her, half smiled, let her eyes roll back into her head until they were only whites, then slumped to the side. We moved her to the floor, and her eyelids fluttered open.

I didn't see Dawit after lunch. It's the end of the day. Biruk and his other senior residents are not around as much as they were before. They are studying for their exams, only working nights, leaving after morning report to sweat over a complicated textbook written in an unfamiliar language.

It is Finot's turn to carry the heaviest weight. For most other doctors, their obligations decline as they become more senior. In an emergency room, like the operating theatre, the most serious cases require skilled hands, ones that know to pull away from a girl's porcelain-white teeth. It's a lifelong practice, passed hand to hand.

I go downstairs, back to the ER, past a courtyard

where people crowd towards specialty clinics. Women in white shawls, some holding babies, stand against the wall, three deep.

I see Finot. She is on duty tonight, and is taking notes about the people scattered about the ER. The bleeding man, the woman with the humming heart. She is nodding as she walks along, pen in hand. The sun is fading, and the windows are turning slowly black, reflecting people watching, waiting.

QR is for Quiet Room.

Near the hospital, coffin sellers line the road. Location, location, location. I try not to take it personally. Beautiful swoops of gold weave over the red felt of a casket. Outside one the shops, a father scoops last night's injera onto his son's plate. Father to son, cradle to grave, even these people, one day, in their beautiful boxes.

A shroud, my mom said to me, when I asked her how she wanted to be buried. Let the worms dig into me straight away.

"Doctor!"

A man pounded on the side of his coffin, showing me how sturdy it was. I nod admiringly.

How did he know I was a doctor?

I keep walking.

The thin metal smell of poorly scrubbed gasoline dissolves into my blood, drives itself deeply into my smallest spaces. Beside me, cars honk, trucks chug. Between them, people flit across the road. At the bottom, the corner where people gather selling tea or fried bread to the long lines queued outside the Ministry of Immigration, three women push past me, smiling, carafes of tea steaming in their hands, run towards a busy bus stopped up the road. I promise myself, as I often do, that one day I'll buy all the bread, so they can go home early, but I never get around to it.

Hospital gate, teams of students walking hand in hand, leaning on each other, laughing. I wave at ones I know, stop a few times to bump shoulders. Near the ER, the high wail of a woman, then I see her, face down in the gravel outside our one open window. She rises to her knees, then throws herself to the ground again.

Her mother. Her father. Her sister. Her daughter.

Abat, I say, and tap the blue-jacketed security guard on the shoulder. His eyes on the woman, he unlatches the emergency's half-door to let me pass. The smell of sickness.

Busy. Busier and busier all the time.

An ultrasound on a young man's heart shows it swinging wildly in a bag of water. Slowly, Finot guides a needle into it, through his flat chest. The patient watches the screen with us, the white metal glinting on the screen, until it sits just next to the collapsing muscle. Finot pulls on the end of the syringe, and it fills with tawny fluid. We drain almost a litre of it, and the fat vessels in his neck flatten. His breathing eases. Ours too.

Ahmed has gone home, vitamins in his pocket. He

stopped bleeding. Providence and some platelets. In his bed, a man with a bad leg, purple to the knee.

Circulation problems. He had it taken from him last night. Today he is bandaged, wincing in pain. I spend a minute studying his remaining foot. It is cool, and at a certain vantage, out of the corner of my eye, there is the faintest bit of blue. He will lose it also, I think, but I don't say so.

A breathless man, found by the road, bruised. He was beaten, or hit by a car. No one knows. We worked on him for long minutes, hoping to get his heart to beat, but his pupils widened, no more use for the light. There were no wails.

I leave the ER ravenous for lunch, and a young man steps in front of me and says, "My muzzer . . . my muzzer . . . ," and points behind me. What about her, I say, and his eyes become wet. He has used all of his English.

She is breathing fast and shallow. Finot's already at the bedside.

"I'm clear," she says, glancing down towards her feet, to make sure her body is not touching the green bed's frame.

"You're clear," she says, turns to the dozen white-coated students ringing the windowless resuscitation room, crowded into the doorway. All kinds of interested eyes for these exciting parts.

"Everyone's clear?" A final warning, and she pushes the button of the electrified paddle she's holding above the old woman's heart pumping too fast to fill.

Whompf. The woman's body jerks, and an arm flies across her torso. Eyes turn to the monitor, but Finot and I put our fingers on each side of the woman's neck, to that spot beside the Adam's apple, where the muscles come together in a Y shape. The pulse is easy to feel. It is 80, regular for now.

"No CPR," I say to the nurse poised on a stool.

"Sorry," I say to Finot, and step back.

She waits for me to continue. I stay quiet.

The woman moans, and an arm rises weakly. Her son steps forward, guides it back down. Her fingers wrap around his.

One learns in the anatomy lab an early lesson. You can pull a human right apart, cut through muscles and fascia to the curved heart, dig through a bucket of swirling feet, pull one out and examine how closely the nerves and tendons run together, but you keep gloves over the hands, because they are so exactly like our own.

The tracing on the monitor jitters as the woman moves. It is one of the last with all its parts. The cables disappear. We aren't sure if patients unhook them when backs are turned or if nurses take them. There is a market for everything.

The woman's daughters hover by the door, in tight jeans, purses dangling from their elbows. A man with a bloody broken leg props himself on his elbow in the room's only other bed, the stretcher a welded metal square we squealed against the wall just moments before to make more room for the crowd. His catheter bag, half full with dark urine, sways from the frame.

The air is stuffy. There are no windows.

"Why do you think she is going in and out of ventricular tachycardia?" Finot asks a junior resident, referring to the fast, unstable rhythm she just short-circuited.

"Infarction? Electrolyte imbalance? Toxicologic?" he answers.

We may never know. This is the third time we've shocked this woman. This morning she was talking. Now, only gasps. She will be dead soon.

The monitor behind us beeps as her heart starts to skip more beats.

"Does anyone in the family speak English?"

The son who stopped me shakes his head, at least knowing that much of it.

Finot replaces the defibrillator paddles in the ancient machine, uses a piece of cotton to wipe the blue gel from the woman's breasts. Two red rectangles the size of a hand are burned into her skin from the current. Finot pulls the dress back to her neck.

"Let's talk in the hall," I say, turning away from the curious faces, the nursing students, the man on his elbow, staring. One of the nurses stays to watch the woman's hands lest she pull at the wires.

In the hall, Finot talks to them in Amharic, her voice trilling softly. A cross shines on her necklace. I can understand nothing, but know what she is saying.

They are rapt. There is no conversation that people attend more closely than this one. She has their complete attention.

This is the end of your mother's life. I'm sad today is that day. Her heart is weak, and we can't keep shocking it like we have. It hurts her, and won't fix what's wrong. It's her time to die. It might be in a few minutes or a few hours. It is good that you are here, to be with her. We will—

A nurse whispers into her ear. Finot listens, nods, and continues. The family stands, staring, the son with his Nokia cell phone in his hand, holding it like a microphone towards her. The hallway is narrow, and people push past, jostling us. Finot speaks more loudly to make her voice heard above the noise.

I have an idea.

I excuse myself, move down the corridor and try the handles on the beaten grey doors that line it. Locked. Locked. Open. A bed on the floor, a window blacked out with newspaper. The night resident's room.

I try another. A group of nurses look up from their lunch.

Locked. Open.

A graveyard of equipment, tubes, machines. The skeletons of charity.

Open. A naked stretcher sits on blocks. Sun beams through the window. Plaster of Paris is matted to the floor. An orthopaedics room, for putting on casts. It's a bit dirty, but . . . I swivel the window wide. The sun is hot on my face, and the air is fresh. In the tree outside, a bird sways on a branch, chirping. With the door shut, the hospital can almost be forgotten. It's a good place to die.

At least, better. I kick pieces of plaster into the middle of the floor, brush off the room's single chair with my hand. A cloud of white dust floats into the air.

We'll move the woman and her family in here, I decide, and leave to find a broom.

Finot has finished with the family, and they are again at the bedside in the yellow resuscitation room, echoing with beeps and a thinning crowd of students whispering to each other, waiting for more shocks. The man with the broken leg winces, his hands on his thigh, trying to turn over, even just a bit. A friend is at his side, helping with one hand; in the other, a plastic bag with rolls of x-rays.

I find a cleaner changing the trash and pull her into the room. I clean the counter while she mops the floor. I take a second chair, abandoned for a moment at a patient's bedside, and place it into the quiet room.

We have a quiet room in Toronto, too, but it's not where people die. It is a place where we put families so we can deliver bad news, where fathers can collapse to the ground in grief, hidden from others. It is windowless, and there is a fake potted plant in the corner. There are enough chairs for eight people.

Between families, porters and cleaners sit with each other on their breaks, laughing, showing each other videos on their phones. When they see a nurse leading a family closer, they sober, leave with bowed heads.

There is no dying room in any hospital I've been in. There should be. My friend Margaret told me about "crying rooms" in the Congo, but those are for patients who need procedures done without anaesthetic. The man in the bloody cast, next door. This was his crying room.

It is nearly clean, the smell of the antiseptic wafting out the window. The door is too narrow for the stretcher she's on. We can use the black plastic mattress she's lying on, carry her in it like a blanket.

I return to the ER's main room, patients coughing, families spooning mouthfuls of stew towards their moms. I find Biruk. He is surrounded by interns, and a worried man with a letter in his hand. I interrupt, tell him my plan, ask him to recruit others. Within a few minutes, six of us are ready to lift. I show them the room. They nod.

Finot returns from some distant floor of the hospital. She and her colleagues are becoming precious commodities even outside the ER. They are able to do ultrasounds, find veins in bleeding patients when others cannot. I tell her to inform the family of the move. She pauses, looks at Biruk, then agrees.

I know that glance. There is reluctance in it. I've learned to watch for it.

A retired physician from Hungary, keen to teach about antibiotics without spending time first at the bedside, pulls residents from their work in the ER to sit in a classroom. A visiting NGO offers an obstetric ultrasound course because it's what they do, and the more seats they fill, the better it looks to their donors, so Finot, on her one weekend off, takes four hours of buses to and from the teaching site, though there are no obstetrical probes on the ultrasound we have, nor does the ER see pregnant women. An academic at a distant university gets grant money that it must spend lest it not get any more, and tells Black Lion what it wants to do instead of asking what needs to be done. She and her colleagues publish papers on their success without African authors. Last week, a neurosurgeon from Holland, old enough to know better, grey hairs poking from beneath his surgical cap, stood in the middle of the ER, taking pictures of himself with sick people he never touched in the background, while Biruk stood at the nursing station, helping a young mother find a way to pay for a CT scan.

I pull the two of them aside. "Is this a good idea?"

They glance at each other. Biruk shrugs.

This means no.

"I thought they would like privacy, away from the many people, the loud machines. You know, that room is clean. It has sunshine. There are some birds."

It sounds foolish now.

"Yes, it's a nice idea," Finot says. "These people, though, they want to know that everything is being done. It is better that she dies that way, otherwise it will seem that we don't care."

The crowd of interns I've gathered is waiting by the door, ready to move the woman, or get back to work.

Biruk says, "If someone sicker comes in who needs the bed, we can move her. But if not, I think Finot is right."

"OK. I understand. Sorry I didn't ask you sooner."

They both nod, and Biruk dismisses the interns, who disperse with some relief.

We decide not to shock her again. Her eyes are closed, her hands loose by her side. We place the mask loosely on her face, and pure oxygen whistles over her mouth. We leave the family at the bedside, glancing up at the monitor every now and again as it beeps with the skips.

I sit behind the nursing station, stomach rumbling, humbled, watching white coats flash behind curtains. It's tough to say I'm proud of these people, as I have had nothing to do with making them. Still, daily, I feel something akin to that when I watch these doctors navigate a floor full of sick and worried people. Maybe it's awe. Maybe that's what pride was supposed to be in the first place: the awe one feels at participating in something beautiful.

S is for system.

We gave the residents their final exams yesterday. Aklilu, Assefu, Sisay, their proud Ethiopian teachers, each of whom, though not having done a residency, understood the alphabet, whom it could help. Janis, an emergency doctor from Wisconsin, an American university devoting themselves to the same work, flew in to join us.

The residents wore suits and dresses. Biruk was first. We shook hands. His palms were sweaty. In the basement classroom, where he had heard so many stories, Janis and I told him one about an imaginary pregnant woman hit by a bus, nearly dead with a baby inside, the same story our teachers told us.

"First I would put her in the trauma area of my emergency . . ."

As if there were such a place. I put a check mark on my answer key.

". . . and attach her to oxygen, monitors, and get a complete set of vital signs . . ."

Looking for cables, scrambling to find a blood pressure cuff that worked. Check.

". . . start two large-bore IVs, running wide open, and call for O negative blood . . ."

Leave the ER, run down the hall to the blood bank, but it's locked, the person away or at home. Check mark.

"What are her vital signs now?" he asked anxiously, an imaginary treatment running in through wide IVs.

"Blood pressure . . . unattainable."

"Does she have a radial pulse?"

"Only a weak femoral."

And then it's gone. No blood, no operating room with a surgeon on the other end of the phone, just you, ultrasound probe in your hand, sweeping the uterus for a second heartbeat while the room slowly fills with nurses, students, the driver, last, the husband in a dirty green jacket, cap in his hand. You can barely move.

". . . I would turn the patient in left lateral decubitus position . . ."

He went on. He answered all our questions, saved her and the baby in a world we've told him about but which he has yet to see. He left the room. Seble sat down, then Sofia, Yenealem.

"I would move the patient to the trauma room . . ."

We played our stone faces, and they left, wondering. Aklilu and I tallied their marks. They all passed. Ethiopia had its first emergency doctors.

At dinner a day later, I stood in front of them, their families, a small gathering of professors and emissaries from the Ministry of Health, in the Ghion's old ballroom, through which Haile Selassie himself once walked, talking about truths half-seen.

"You might think that emergency medicine is about the skills you've learned in resuscitation, grace under pressure, or how to read an electrocardiogram. It's not. It's about a room that never closes . . ."

They listened, the weight of ninety million people not yet fully felt.

Biruk and Sofia were to remain at Black Lion; Sebleh and Yenealem, to return to their home cities, try to grow emergency rooms there.

I looked at each of their faces in turn. This was a big day, a milestone after many tries. Why weren't we more glad? I shifted, uncomfortable in my seat. A truth, obscured by this day, moved into view.

Who would save *them*?

When I knew enough about airways that I could be left alone, all that remained was finding an ER with hours to fill. The nurses were there, the drugs, specialists waiting for my call. I showed up, grabbed some charts, an interchangeable part of an articulating system, sweeping people through. If it wasn't me, it would work as well with someone else who knew what I did.

In Ethiopia, not a single person outside of this dim room knew what these four doctors were capable of.

Nor could they show it yet. There were places where they could outside of the country, places where they would be paid five times what they would be here, maybe even ten. Rwanda, floating with NGOs funded in dollars or euros by governments trying to reconcile standing idly when they were needed most. Botswana, and its diamond mines. By leaving, they could pull their families up, allow them to take taxis instead of walking along the side of the road at night. Worldwide, money sent home through Western Union eclipses foreign aid and, with none of it perpetuating jobs for foreigners or hiding secondary agendas, does more to alleviate poverty.

Today, as always, the future wobbled, uncertain. It listed with lives of people I had come to care about. Which way would it fall?

I can see two ways. One, on this dry autumn day, after many attempts and much adversity, it tips with the weight of two men and two women who know better than anyone, perhaps anywhere, what it takes to save lives lost in a country with modest means. As important as their knowledge is their vantage, at the edge of a tide of people, poor and sick and afraid, because they see, perhaps too clearly, what it takes—the number of surgeons, how much blood, what type of immunizations, the pounds of plaster for all the busted bones and the pairs of crutches to bear them.

Some stay in the ER and are given autonomy to make small improvements, day by day. The chance to make things better, for themselves and their patients, even a bit, adds enough to their small salary to make it a life worth leading. Though the birr they earn are not enough to travel, they can live, take a week off here and there, leave work on time most days. The women talk to the female residents about how to have children, be an ER doctor, and stay well. Students start to show up on time for morning report, some even skipping lunch to learn, stomachs growling. Sofia wins a teaching award.

Some learn the language of science, how to calculate p-values and numbers needed to treat, download the few papers from others writing about a similar road, connect with them, avoid their mistakes, publish their own papers. A resident project, mapping out places in the city where pedestrians are hit, allows for speed bumps, then roadside lights, finally a pedestrian boulevard. The rate of head injuries requiring surgery falls.

An international campaign to prevent rheumatic disease is funded after Gelaw and Aklilu show how many young years and millions of birr are lost to it. Encouraged, Demelesh, with the Ministry of Health, publishes national consensus guidelines on how best to manage heart attacks when money is scarce. People who suffer them return to their jobs driving steamrollers, pounding pavement flat. The guidelines, containing only generic drugs, are useful not just in Addis but in Asmara. Juba. Nairobi. Vientiane. Toronto. Companies that distribute essential medicines thrive, eat into profits of those who bank only on the rich. Borders blur.

More ER's open in Addis, then in other Ethiopian cities with medical universities, then the countryside, then the camps where people huddle drinking black water. They are all connected, nodes in an emerging network. From necessity, the ecological footprints are small, greatly efficient. No water is wasted.

Nurses linger longer in the ER, some making it a life's career. They face burnout, and some learn how to address it. Having more eyes in the ER means cables stay on the monitors, and the ones that break are noticed and repaired the same day. A local economy emerges around the buzzing activity the ER holds.

South Africans with ultrasounds to sell sponsor a yearly conference. An Ethiopian pharmaceutical company, part of an intra-African consortium, produces a new drug for leishmaniasis. Two twenty-year-old medical bioengineers, one from Dar es Salaam, one from Addis, develop a 3-D cervical collar printed from old tires.

The residency grows. Demand is high. Soon, a second program is needed in Addis. A third. Demelesh opens a fourth in Hawassa, a day's drive away. The graduates are experts in a new field, one that matters to 80 per cent of the world. More students see jobs in their own country. They stay.

Two years of tense peace in Juba, and the medical university there, the only one in South Sudan, sends its best graduate to Addis. After a four-week intensive Amharic course, she begins a one-year fellowship in emergency medicine systems. Biruk and Finot, hair greying, are among her many teachers. Once her year is finished, she returns to South Sudan and is able to start an emergency department of her own and, using Addis's curriculum, a residency.

Biruk, Finot, Gelaw, Gemechis form the first team of teachers from Addis Ababa University, help her deliver lectures, then give the first set of exams to students as nervous as they once were. They tell the story of that pregnant lady walking home at night, hit by a car. The next year, they make up their own. Ayen applies for a scholarship to attend.

In Juba's emergency room, the cables disappear, some of the nurses quit, but they treat everybody, Dinka, Nuer, Christian, Muslim, sickest first, then everyone else in the order they come. I am old, and can no longer travel. Sebleh visits Toronto with her grandchildren.

A waiter at my side. I hold my glass towards him.

Another version is a future that budges but does not tip, the weight stacked so heavily against these four, and their country's ambition, that even with five more, then six, it follows the past's worn track, and the ERs they return to remain the same as before. Their salaries, the long duties, the problems with the oxygen tanks. As more people arrive to the city, the ER gets busier, more overcrowded, and the poor are even more tightly crammed. More private hospitals open, and Black Lion, already straining to help the few it can, loses more doctors and nurses to them.

As before, people wait days to have their broken bones stabilized, and on the rare day they are finally seen, by a tired surgeon, already overworked by her six jobs, they are sent back to the ER to be cared for by Biruk and Finot. Although they know emergency medicine, they don't have a chance to do it much. Their skills fade with the world we helped them imagine.

The ER remains an undeveloped notion rather than a place as important as an airway. Donors drop off more used or out-of-date equipment that works for a week or a year, then gets thrown out. Students arrive unannounced from all over the world, then leave early to go to the market and buy scarves. The crooked door in the learning centre loses another wheel, gets stuck while a class is inside, and needs to be shaken from the track to free them. It is stowed under the stairwell, with that old grey desk and the chair with a broken seat.

Some of the graduates start missing days. Parents now, they need to make money somewhere. Some persist for a while in the public system, enticed by the possibility, but as community dwindles, their motivation does too. The salary remains too small to live on in a city where the rich grow fast and their commute becomes longer and longer. Applications for the emergency medicine residency fall as prospective students see little hope for a paying career.

A few emergency rooms start here and there, their doors held open by universities across the world, but the flow between them never quite starts.

Medical studies continue to focus mostly on how to squeeze out another person in a thousand at tremendous cost, rather than on how best to spread what is already available to as many people as possible. Guidelines are paid for by drug companies, and medicine and money wind so tightly together, you can barely see the difference. A healthy year of a Canadian's life is assessed at $60,000. New guidelines suggest resuscitating infants as early as twenty-one weeks.

People cling to borders, place their children on white plastic sheets outside tent hospitals claimed by NGOs flying a variety of flags. Their doctors visit Addis on their R & R sometimes, talk about how cosmopolitan it is. Inequity grows in the region. Even Addis becomes tense. The University of Toronto halts flights for faculty, just for now, the provost says. Legal issues.

The woman in Juba University learns some emergency medicine from a few doctors who visit twice a year, though rarely the same person twice. They teach her about the airway, how to intubate, resuscitate, defibrillate, but there is an outbreak of violence and disease in a more strategically important country. Visitors become few. Her back hallway is lined with malarious men and bleeding women. She sees as many as she can, but it's hard to keep track of them all. A cousin suggests she join him in America. He can find her a job. One day, she's gone.

Now, in the ballroom, Aklilu and Sisay say some final words, call to the front all the partners who have hastened this day. Everyone is standing. The deputy minister, phone in one hand, shakes my hand. We all pose for a group photo.

On a wall, projected images of times past flicker. The ER without curtains, these four young doctors standing awkwardly in the middle of it.

T is for tikur.

Last days. I am ceding my apartment to a Canadian who is helping Addis Ababa University grow family medicine. His may be an even longer road.

I walk slowly down the stairs, notice new cracks, a plant wilting in a window. When change is near, unnoticed details grow clear. Outside, on the cobblestone street, men pass bricks hand to hand, while two others spin a churning drum, cement spattered on their bare backs.

Morning report has been quieter without the graduates. Sofia and Biruk have yet to report for duty, taking some weeks off to rest, consider their future. We glance at their empty chairs. The newest residents have yet to start. I have heard there are five men and women, from all over the country.

The residents hosted a party for me last week, in the learning centre. They came from the ER, from ophthalmology and orthopaedics rotations, stethoscopes and reflex hammers in their white coats, brought a cake with white icing, my name written in red. They had signed a card with their names and kind words. I tried to skirt sentiment, and almost did.

I talked about how brave they were, to be standing at the bedside in the middle of the night, unprotected, and at times, unsupported, but that if they weren't there, the person in the bed, sick and poor, would have no one at all, and they didn't . . .

I needed to stop.

. . . didn't choose either of those fates, you know, but to have you next to them, working to meet their suffering, even if you can't, is perhaps the last act of kindness they will know.

I finished. Barely. I promised to be back soon.

The residents drifted to their work, one by one. Gelaw and Gemechis lingered, stacked plates with me, placed chairs back behind desks. Talk turned from my plans to theirs, the challenges that remained. The poor pay, the meagre supplies, the struggle for recognition from their peers as a specialist. I told them that of all the differences I had seen in the past years, their attention to these problems was the most crucial one. With it, and time, they will dissolve.

"It's true. That's the good news."

"What's the bad news?" Gemechis asked.

I smiled. "There's a bigger one behind it." They laughed. "Hey, are you guys on call this weekend?"

They shook their heads.

"I had an idea . . ."

We met this morning, and with Yonas, a nurse who had heard our plan, filled buckets with water and soap, pushed patient beds away from walls, winced with them as the bag of sand dangling off the foot of their bed, pulling their fractured leg to length, rocked to a stop. Under the grime and bacteria, clean white tiles emerged.

Gelaw stood on a ladder, slid a Plexiglas cover and its years of dust from a skylight, handed it down. Yonas and I dipped old newspapers in blue washing fluid and wiped away the smudges.

Gelila was the senior resident in the emergency department, tending the sickest. She shook her head as she passed by. "You guys are crazy," she said happily, grateful for the company.

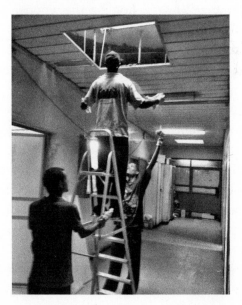

It was calm in the ER. Though it held the same number of cases as usual, there were fewer family members than on weekdays, no packs of whispering students.

"So you are leaving us soon," Gelila said, joining us, trying to scrape a sticker from the wall, its logo long faded.

"Tomorrow."

"It means a lot to us, you know. That you came and stayed."

"It does to me too."

"And you're coming back?"

"Yes."

Circles of soap streaked the glass.

A nurse interrupted, and Gelila left us. A few minutes later, she returned while Gemechis and I repositioned the ladder under the second skylight.

"Dr. James, can I ask you about a patient?"

"Of course," I said, holding the wooden frame so Gelaw could climb.

"A fifty-year-old woman from outside Addis presents with easy bruising and fatigability." Everything's low. Platelets too.

"Visit hematology clinic on Monday," Gelaw said from above, smiling, and handed me the square sheet of plastic.

We discussed some other possibilities, infections or cancers, Gelaw sitting on the ladder's lowest rung. I could tell by what Gelila had already ordered that she'd thought about these things. It was just good to have someone to talk to.

A nurse at her arm again. Gemechis and I flipped the clear cover over, started wiping the other side.

After an afternoon of work, our fingers bleached and stinging, we stood at triage, looking into the ER with our hands on each other's shoulders. Light streamed through the ceiling, and the smell of sickness was cut, at least for a few hours, with a sharp one of ammonia. It was good. Maybe even something to believe in.

"OK," Yonas said, clapped his hands. "I must go home."

Sure, sure, us too, we all said, the reverie broken. We grabbed our bags and set off in separate directions.

I passed the hospital gate. A guard, toothpick in his mouth, smiled, half stood as I walked by, then sat back down. Music played from the mobile phone in his hand. No one waited.

The tent home was shuttered. At the bottom of the hospital hill, cars idled, chugging black smoke. A police officer stood in front of them, and with a shrill whistle, waved the whining line forward.

A crowd of kids kicked a ball back and forth in an empty parking lot. It rolled towards me and I swiped at it poorly, caught the edge, and it stuttered to the side. They raced.

I turned towards the Piassa, the old town, where I'd been staying, my mind running through planes and times. My backpack was heavy with papers and books, so I stopped, let it drop from my shoulder, put it between my legs, kneaded the muscles in my neck.

I looked back the way I had come. The boys playing football, the police officer sweating in his uniform, a crowd clustered at the tea corner, talking, selling belts and passport covers.

I am leaving this place.

Why did I come?

Beside me, in the shade of a building, people tilt back on red chairs, drinking coffee, watching the same scene.

I sit.

A woman in a white dress approaches with a clay coffee pot and a tray of cups. She has tattoos on her neck and forehead, like the woman Demelesh sent to the ICU.

She died there yesterday. I'm glad we did everything.

"Buna. Tikur." Coffee. Black.

She pours me a small glass. Green herbs float to the top.

More children have joined the game. The speed has picked up. Some of them wear the same striped shirt, part of a team. A second match breaks out on the side, between the youngest. Their ball is ragged, almost flat. A shot sails high, lands on the cement with a thud.

A charge to the fence. Its chain clangs as bodies bump the corrugated metal. On the other side, an obelisk, a hundred feet high, in homage to soldiers, some who came from as far away as Cuba to fight and die.

These two things, pulling back and forth, fastened together forever. Building up, tearing apart.

I talked to my friend Ian on the phone. Jubilee planning. I told him I was writing a book about emergencies as a sign of life taking care of itself, but wasn't sure where it would go.

"Remember when you told me about that woman in Sudan who walked for two days with a baby's arm sticking from her?"

"Yeah. It was blue."

"Just write about what she was walking towards."

I turn my chair. Black Lion's silhouette cuts the horizon.

There is another place in Addis to which such women walk, some from as far away as Sudan. Addis Ababa Fistula Hospital, also known as the Hamlin Hospital for its Australian founder. I didn't know about it back then, or I would have tried to get that woman there. She had a fistula, a perforation that develops between the vagina and bladder or rectum after labouring, unattended, for days. The baby often dies inside, like hers did, or just after birth, but the pushing wears a hole in the woman. Urine or feces trickle out of her vagina, and she is moved to shacks behind her family's house, laid on hard boards so waste doesn't run down her legs. Over the years, I've seen a few. The holes were so very small, but through them, a future fell. The husband moves on, takes another wife, and the woman is cared for by sisters and friends until she dies.

In some towns, though, I suppose, word of Hamlin Hospital is carried mouth to mouth, and one day, in the middle of the night or the hot of the day, these women are borne towards the place where those small holes can be fixed, and their lives restored. Some arrive with their knees contracted into angles because they haven't moved for a year. Often malnourished and sick, they are nursed until they are well enough to endure an operation, then taught to walk again. Once they can, most never return home. Many of them continue to work at the hospital. The key surgeon is a former patient from 1962 who never went to medical school but assisted in so many fistula surgeries, she started doing them. She is now the best in the world. Of all the many wonders I have seen, it is the single greatest place. Every spot seems like the right one at which to fall to your knees.

I don't read much about her, that woman, the Ethiopian one. Mamitu. I found only one article, in the *New York Times*. I wonder why. It's a powerful story. Maybe she likes it quiet. The Australian founder is much easier to find.

I swivel again. On the hill opposite Black Lion, a rose-roofed hotel claims a whole hill. There, tall men with white gloves tip top hats and hold the door, and inside, ceilings soar. A woman plays piano next to a display of pastries and chocolate cakes, children tumble past paintings thirty feet high. I visit sometimes to find quiet space, or have a glass of wine. You could be anywhere in the world.

The distance between the two places is not one just any person can cover by walking. Lifetimes. Maybe not at all. My privilege offers me that ignorance, the advantage of not needing to know what stands in the way. To someone with fewer means, different sex or skin or tribe, they know. No matter how I might try, I can't even tell what walls I'm missing.

Another striped shirt joins the boys. The kids with the mohawks are watching, arms crossed, cardboard box leaning against their legs.

I met one of them last week. Well, he's a man now. He shared my table at the busy restaurant where I go to take lunch.

"Doctor?" he asked, noticing the stethoscope in my bag.

"Yes. You?"

"Businessman. But I once was that boy," he said, pointing out the window at a child with rags for clothes.

His father died, then his mother. He moved to the streets, made a living however he could, selling food, sometimes taking it. One day, he crossed a line he shouldn't have and went to jail.

"I became a violent man," he said, studying his scarred hands.

He was in solitary confinement for two years, threatened every day with being killed. He believed it.

Someone taught him to read, then he got a radio, learned English from BBC.

"I began to study psychology," he said, "what made a man. I started to know myself, and slowly, I changed. I discovered that though my past was part of me, my future was mine to claim. I grew less angry. They let me out of my chains."

His death sentence was commuted to life in jail, and he started to work in the prison, organizing activities so inmates wouldn't be idle. Violence fell. The wardens noticed, and he was transferred to another jail to accomplish something similar. In 2000, on the eve of the Ethiopian millennium, the president pardoned thousands of prisoners who had shown reform.

"And just like that"—the man snapped his fingers— "I was released. Jail was better than Oxford would have been for me because I decolonized my mind," he said, tapping his head with a finger.

He had set himself free.

He stood, put his coat over his shoulders.

"Thanks for sharing your table."

I sat, dumb. Another teacher. I was an hour late returning to the ER. When there was a quiet moment, I asked some students if racism was as common in Ethiopia as it was in North America. No, no, they shook their heads, not at all. Muslims, Christians, side by side. Sometimes we don't even know. What about people from Gambella, the ones who look Sudanese? I heard someone once say that they weren't real Ethiopians. The residents looked at each other, tittered nervously.

Rich and poor, young and old, black and blacker. The mind's dividing lines. If there are none, it makes judgements anyway. Evidence shows that in American ERs, black people receive less pain medicine. This is even true of children with appendicitis. They are offered less, out of some mistaken belief by a doctor or nurse that though the appendix is always in the exact same place, people with different skin tone experience pain differently. The same is true of the elderly. The deepest sadness is that with time, people forget that relief is something they can ask for, that their comfort matters as much as anyone's.

What is true in the ER is true of the world that made it. In our time, it appears we get to take a continent's riches, then pretend we are doing them a favour by helping them with poverty.

If we can make the time, that is. People seem to be getting tired of the argument that the walking woman deserves the same privileges they have, if they ever believed it. But now I have a growing sense of a new counterargument being offered. It is that with all the ecological ruin we've sown, she is simply too late to the party. Sorry but we're just tidying up. They don't understand that what they shut down to believe that lie is exactly what is needed both to meet that woman, and to cure what ails us.

What she was walking towards was never a place. It was a direction towards a world that made sense.

The arm. Blue.

So fucked up.

The street beside me starts to blur.

Shadows slant. In the parking lot, the game has stopped. One of the striped boys holds the ball under his arm, talking to a friend. The street boys have moved on.

I sit forward, let my elbows rest on the table, and look around. A man with a thin moustache, in a grey overlarge suit, teal tie, waits, his plastic-bag briefcase on the table. The young waitress, leg up on a concrete step, counts her money, then puts it back in the black belt around her waist, raises one arm to the sky, stretches, tendons on the back of her hands pulling taut like wires. For a moment, I see it all, then it's gone.

U is for urban.

I've always wondered if, before you die, there's a sign. A vision, or a sound. There is a tone on my phone I use only when I'm on trauma call. It tells me someone has been hurt. When I hear it, my heart shoots to a hundred, just like theirs.

Ring . . . ringring. Riiiiiinnnng.

I roll over in bed towards the bright screen. A message to call switchboard. I pick up the hotel phone, tap in the digits.

"Dr. Maskalyk, trauma team leader. Yes, I'll hold."

I stand, move the thick curtain to the side. Below me, the bright letters of St. Mike's emergency room. No palm tree. The woopwoopwoop of a helicopter gets louder.

"Never mind . . . I hear it," I say and hang up.

I hop into my pants, one leg, the other, throw on my scrub top, grab my hospital badge, walk briskly to the elevator, press "ground."

I've started doing trauma shifts in addition to my emergency ones. It's exciting, and I get to spend more than five minutes with a person. It took Ethiopia to remind me how much I liked that. And what I learn in the trauma room, I'll take back to Black Lion.

It has been proved that both money and lives are saved if a few hospitals are equipped to handle specific conditions. Strokes, heart attacks. The same is true of injuries. In the dark floors below, we have floors of nurses who tend only to the wounded, operating rooms at the ready with surgeons nearby, and experienced physicians like me to make sure a hurt person survives long enough to meet them. St. Mike's is one of only two places in this city that handles the injuries that happen when bodies collide.

The more people that get hurt, and the worse they are injured, the more I get paid. It's a strange job.

I'm supposed to be less than twenty minutes away from the hospital, but I'm staying even closer, right across the street. It is the first five minutes that are the most exciting.

On the street. It is around midnight, and the air is damp, filled with invisible seeds of spring. I jog down the sidewalk, cut the light, up the hospital ramp. I flash my badge on the door and it beeps open. The entire trauma team is already in the room. Anaesthesia, orthopaedics, general surgery, x-ray, and respiratory technicians, two ER nurses, one from the trauma ICU, a handful of medical students, a chaplain.

"Scoot, scoot," one of the nurses is saying to a grey-haired man huddled under a blanket on the ambulance stretcher, two red units of blood held high on posts above him. An air medic is holding his IV tubing so it doesn't get crossed while a portable monitor taps out a regular rhythm. He shuffles from their narrow bed to the hard trauma one.

I got a call about him a couple of hours ago, from a hospital an hour outside the city. A transfer. He was at the bar minding his own business, an activity associated with a very high risk for winding up in the trauma room, and was punched in the stomach. He tried to sleep it off, but the pain wouldn't quit, so he went to the nearest hospital. An emergency doctor miles away scanned his abdomen, saw intestines floating in blood, and called a toll-free number that connected the two of us. We talked about the case, what he'd already done to help him. We decided to give the man more clotting factor, send him our way with blood.

I glance at a crimson hanging bag. It is still full, the cells only trickling in. The IVs in his hands are too small.

The man props himself on his elbows, grimacing. The blanket falls away. His belly appears swollen.

"Sir, I'm Dr. Maskalyk. You're at St. Michael's Hospital. We're here to take care of you. There are going to be a lot of things happening at once."

I put my hand on his stomach, near his belly button. It is tense. I push gently, then let go. His face twists with a flash of pain. It's called rebound tenderness, an abdomen inflamed by blood or infection. It nearly always means an operation.

"Sir, open your mouth," the anaesthetist says.

The surgical resident squirts a stream of blue gel onto the man's belly. "Sorry! Cold," she says brightly.

A nurse affixes EKG leads to his chest.

The x-ray tech points at the hanging x-ray machine, then at his own chest. I shake my head.

An orthopaedic resident is feeling along the man's legs for fractures. "Tell me if it hurts anywhere."

"Do you know where you are?"

"Any allergies?"

"Another poke . . . Poke!" A nurse juts in a larger IV. The man winces.

Simon, my emergency doctor colleague and friend, opens the trauma room door.

"Heard you were in here. You need another set of hands?"

"No, man, I'm good."

"OK. Welcome back."

"Thanks."

"Fentanyl?" a nurse asks, suggesting something for pain. I turn behind, look at the big yellow numbers of his blood pressure and heart rate. Pressure is 85. Heart rate 110. Too low. Too high.

"Let's wait."

The resident manoeuvres the probe on the man's belly. The screen is mostly dark, with a few bright patches. The black is blood. It looks worse than what was described to me over the phone.

"We have a larger IV, so let's squeeze the blood in with the Level 1," I say, referring to the pneumatic compressor that can empty a bag in seconds.

"Don't you want to use ours?" she asks.

"No. This is good."

She frowns. Our blood is passed hand to hand, two nurses checking it at each stage to be sure the right person gets the right type.

I'm not throwing this away. It says "O" right on it. Let me tell you a story about a shivering man.

An orderly pulls a heated blanket from our warmer, drapes it over the patient's legs.

"You're going to be okay, sir," I say as the bags are put into the clear cask of the compressor.

The trauma room phone rings. It's Najma, the trauma surgeon. I tell her about the ultrasound. She'll meet the man in the OR.

"Now we can shoot that chest," I say to the x-ray technician. He moves his cantilevered machine into place, slides a metal negative into a slot in the trauma stretcher.

"X-ray!" he shouts, and those of us without the patterned lead aprons duck behind those who wear them.

"Do you want the massive transfusion protocol?" a nurse asks.

"One sec," I say, turn away, glance through the guidelines. Near the bottom: *blunt trauma, ongoing hypotension.* "Let's do it."

She picks up the phone. "Hi, blood bank, it's Alaina, a nurse in the trauma room . . ."

A surgery resident and I huddle around the x-ray machine's display, shielding the bright fluorescent lights. Looks good. A porter arrives with a red cooler, full of blood, frozen plasma and platelets. We put the box on the man's bed, click up the side rails, then roll him to the row of elevators just down the hall, wires from the portable monitor trailing to the side.

I see Laura, the ER doctor in major. She waves. Soon, she will tell Simon fifteen short stories about a person's worst day.

The elevator door slides open and we pack it full. On the fourth floor, a nurse in scrubs and a blue bonnet greets us, takes the chart from my hands, and pushes the bed past a green line on the floor that marks the threshold of the operating rooms. I can go no farther in my dirty shoes.

"Goodbye, sir."

I ride the elevator down with a nurse from the ER. She shows me pictures of a daughter on her phone.

"Time for you to get one," she says, rubbing her chin, pointing out the white bristles in my beard.

"I know."

I pass through the ER. It is after one now, and those who needed to be pushed up the tilted sidewalk have limped out. The rest are in hospital beds, glancing at the monitors beside them, wondering at the numbers. A few nod in the waiting room, a dozen or so still at home, deciding whether they can sleep through the night with the pain in their back, the voices in their head.

I leave the hospital, cross the park, looking for food. It's breakfast time in Addis. A man sleeps slumped against the church doors. A man with a speaker blaring from the back of his BMX bike rides in circles, high on crystal. You learn how to tell. It's different than crack. Much more focused.

Store fronts are dark. Bright lights stream onto the sidewalk from a falafel shop a block away, but a man has stacked their last chairs onto a table, and is swirling water on the vinyl floor.

Shouldn't go too far. I turn around, walk back to my hotel, past pawn shops dangling guitars behind metal bars.

I buy a bag of chips from the machine in the hotel lobby, and it drops from its spinning rack. I eat them in bed, flicking through a hundred channels, before turning off the light.

Ring . . . ringring. Riiiiiinnnng.

My phone glows.

STAB WOUND. VITAL SIGNS ABSENT. 5 MINUTES.

I run.

A woman, shielding her boyfriend, was stabbed in the chest by a knife meant for him. Simon is already in the room, ultrasound peering into her chest.

"Any cardiac activity?" I ask as I pull a waterproof gown from the shelf, a pair of gloves, a plastic face shield to stop the spattering blood I'm about to see.

"Can't see any," he says, frowning, adjusting the curved probe.

"IV access?" Snap, one glove. Snap, a second.

"Nope."

A surgery resident stands near the woman's chest, his washed hands held high in the air as if he was in the operating room, ready to cut.

"What year are you?"

"Four."

"Open her chest."

He takes up a scalpel, draws a thin line through her skin, just under her breast, tracing the rib. Yellow fat bursts from its centre.

"Push the tube all the way down," I say to the anaes-thetist at the head of the bed. The tube naturally travels down the less oblique path, into the right side of the tra-chea, deflates the left lung, gives more room for us to see a bleeding heart, which in this bad scenario is the best thing you can hope for.

Simon and I set up at different places on her body, me at her neck, him in her leg, trying to thread a needle into a vein we can't see but know is there. No matter what we find in the chest, she needs a way to get blood, or she'll stay dead. A flash of purple beads into the hub of my syringe as a I poke under her collarbone, but it stops. The veins are flat and empty, hard to cannulate.

Opposite me, the surgery resident makes a cut between her ribs. A litre of blood spills onto the floor. He puts in the rib spreaders, attaches the ratchet.

Clickclickclick. He pulls her chest apart.

"I've got one," Simon says.

"Me too," I say, as I pull back hard on the syringe. Blood floods into its clear barrel.

"Blood," I say, holding up my right hand, my left hold-ing fast the thin line in her subclavian vein. A nurse places IV tubing into it. I don't even look. I twist the two pieces together, sew them to her skin. The Level 1 pump starts humming, squeezing bag after bag into her groin, her neck. The nurses called for blood before I'd even arrived.

I walk around the stretcher. The resident has already put a vascular clamp over a gash in the right ventricle. The muscle is slowly writhing, turning, but not beating. He is massaging it with his palms. A thumb could push right through a human heart.

As the muscle gets its first taste of blood, the twisting becomes smoother, then a thrash. Thrash. Thrash. Thrashthrashthrashthrash.

"I can feel a carotid pulse," the anaesthetist says from above.

"She has a femoral," Simon says.

Her chest is held open by the spreaders, one lung a deflated pink bag. The surgery resident takes his hands from inside her chest. The clamp clangs on the side of the stretcher with each beat.

Clang clang clang clang . . .

He just felt a heart come alive in his hands.

"I need a drain in the right chest . . ." I say, in case the knife cut that far. An ER resident smears iodine on her right breast.

We decide to try and sew the heart, but every time he takes the clamp off to try, with each bound, blood squirts in thin streams, like a lawn sprinkler. Forget it. It can be fixed in the operating room.

The bottoms of my shoes are sticking to the ground. I look down. Blood traces the circles we've made.

We shoot an x-ray, repeat the ultrasound. There is a bit of blood in her abdomen too, but not much, and none coming from the tube in her right chest. It all poured from her heart.

Najma arrives in her hospital greens, surgical bonnet still on.

"What are you waiting for?" she says. "Let's go."

We push the stretcher to the elevator, pulling poles of blood, the anaesthetist at the head of the bed, squeezing the bag. The doors open, and the bed rolls into the white light.

Clang clang clang.

The doors shut.

Silence.

On the ground floor, in the quiet room, I talk to two of the woman's brothers hiding in their hoods, the tangy smell of marijuana clinging to them. One of them has a tattoo tear. They seethe, beside their weeping mother.

Two police stand outside the door, look up from their phones as I leave.

"How is she?" one of them asks.

"Sick, man."

"I've never seen anything like that."

"Yeah, with the chest just open wide that way," says the other. "Looked like an animal. She going to live?"

"Hard to say. There was no blood to her brain for all those minutes. There's a chance, though. Heart's alive."

"So, critical condition, with life-threatening injuries?"

"Exactly," I say. "Catch the guy?"

"Nope."

"Better hurry. I think people are looking for him, and I want to go to bed."

The big one yawns. His partner writes my name on the pad of paper in his hand, then goes into the quiet room.

I pass a TV in the foyer. Already, news of the stabbing, a reporter, live in front of St. Mike's. I take a different door, see the white van with a satellite dish on top, reporter brushing his hair back with his hand.

It's late now, 4 a.m. The night has recovered winter's chill. A paper cup rolls down the blank street. I enter the lobby of the hotel. A man behind the counter looks up. His name tag says "Addis." I say my few words of Amharic. Peace. Hello. How are you. He smiles.

We talk about Ethiopia, how much it's changing. The cranes. Internet. Direct flights.

Emergency doctors, I tell him. He doesn't seem properly impressed. I ride the elevator alone, undress in my room, pull the stiff, unfamiliar sheets over me. Thoughts clatter over one another.

Have I locked the door?

I climb out of bed, check it. Locked.

The air conditioning rattles.

I check my phone.

Is that a siren? No. Whine of the elevator.

Through the thin hotel walls, I can hear a TV.

Who the hell is up at this time?

Ring . . . ringring. Riiiiiinnnng.

Fuck me.

Five a.m.

"Dr. Maskalyk . . ."

Addis is at his computer. He glances up. I don't stop.

Drunk man, found on the sidewalk. No one's sure whether he fell or was assaulted. Many hands hold him down. He has a cut on his forehead, little else.

"Many things are going to happen at once, sir."

I give him a sedative, so he settles. I'm tired. I scan his whole body, take him back to the ER to sober up. Same cops.

"You got some kind of bad luck charm, Doc?" the little one asks.

"I'm starting to think it's you. That guy come with any ID?"

"Nothing."

"All right. Well, he's in bed six. Minor injuries so far. Give us a couple hours."

"Perfect," he says, smiling. "That's not us. That's day shift." He puts his notepad away.

I check on the stab-wound woman in the ICU. She's still intubated. She'll be like that for days. I look through her notes. She got twelve units of blood in the trauma room, ten or so more in the OR. Platelets, plasma too. Heart rate and blood pressure are good. Too soon to say what is left in her brain, what withered during those pulseless minutes. She's got a decent chance. Her body is so young, it might pull the whole thing back together.

The morning shift of nurses is getting handover. My shift is over too. Someone else's phone will chime when a person falls. I change my ringtone.

Addis is at his computer, as bleary as me, waiting for relief. I ask for a late checkout. The elevator opens, and I stand aside for the group of men and women, tapping on their phones, starting their day, then ride up alone. The sheets are twisted from my light sleep, and I move to the window to draw the shade. I linger for a bit, watching the street.

Below me, pigeons fight over scraps. Charnel ground. People crowd mutely at street corners, half asleep. A man leans out his car window, yelling at a cyclist.

I pull the thick curtain closed. I turn on the TV. Aleppo is being bombed to the ground. Migrants are drowning trying to reach Rome. Studies suggest eating kale staves off dementia. Nanoparticles block obesity in mice. Blink. Nuclear deal struck. Baseball player tests positive for steroids. Oil falls. Blink. A dog saves a woman's life. A famous person gets married. Blink. A monk sets himself on fire. Aung San Suu Kyi, freed. Protests in the street.

V is for vertigo.

I talked with my grandfather. First the weather, then the lake. Turns out the cormorants are picking it clean.

"But how are *you* doing?"

"I'm kaput. No good at all. I just get dizzy, you know? My knees hurt, OK, but every now and again, I just get these spells and almost fall."

My mom and dad visited him last weekend. They tried to get him to see a doctor in town. No, he said, I'll wait for Jim. He'll know what to do.

He's waiting for me.

Falling is what got my grandmother. She would be putting the salad bowl away, reaching for the second shelf, and in a blink, she'd be on the floor, orange splinters of glass scattered around her. Or she would pedal back into the sharp edge of a chair. Once, down a couple of stairs.

My grandfather was scared to let her more than reaching distance from him. Like they did when they were courting, they walked arm in arm. He would say, "Now, Katherine, you just stay put until I get back from the garage," but she never could sit still. One day, when he was out of the room, she toppled, cracked her back hard, broke a vertebra, a couple of ribs. He took her to the ER for the last time.

She was never much for eating, and one afternoon, in the hospital, she stopped altogether. Everything she took down would come back up a minute later. She became delirious, talking to people who weren't there. I sat at my kitchen table while a young doctor, in a quiet room a thousand miles away, talked with my family on speaker phone.

"We could put a tube in her stomach," the doctor said. "It would allow us to get some nutrition into her . . . maybe whatever is causing her to get sick will calm down."

"What do you think, Mike?" my mother asked my grandfather, her voice clear and serious.

"I . . . I don't think so . . . Jim? Are you there?"

"Yeah. I'm here."

"Do you think it will help much?"

"No. I don't think it will. I think she's dying, Grandpa."

He could tell.

"OK, then . . . OK, no more tubes."

"I understand," the doctor said, quick to answer, full of relief. "We'll keep the intravenous going for now and maybe she'll turn around." He started talking about medicines that might calm her stomach.

"Thanks, Jim," my dad said, hung up the phone.

He called me a week later. I was on the road. We decided to stop the intravenous, she said. I'll come home now, I answered, knowing she would be dead in a few days.

I gave a eulogy, my second that year. My little brother stood beside me, brave, said his own words, his two children in the front row, too young to understand. We stayed in the church until everyone left, walked my grandfather to my parents' car, then packed up plates of pickles, folded the chairs. In the bright afternoon, the two of us walked out on the frozen lake, and with a hatchet, chipped skins of ice from holes someone had bored a day before.

We lay flat on the snow, looked as far as we could towards the bottom, watching for a fish's white belly. Thirty years before, there would have been nothing else but the blackness below. No funerals, no children. We caught nothing, not even a bite.

Now, my grandfather is about to fall. I asked him some questions, but it's a tough experience to describe.

"I just get dizzy. That's it."

"Is the room spinning?"

"Not much. Just something's not right. I'm old, that's it."

He's had his pacemaker checked. His blood pressure isn't too low. I'm wondering if it's vertigo. That's a skewing of our sixth sense, our position in space. The corrections are so automatic, you don't notice it until it's gone. Our head tilts, and our eyes jerk and come to rest in an instant, before our brain can even sense the gap, and our experience of being in the middle of everything seems continuous. If there is a disconnect, our impression of where we are differs from the actual. We are no longer in contact with the tight shifting line between left and right, up and down. We are lost.

Often, it is the fluid in our inner ear that gets stuck. All vertebrates have this. Fish, birds, dogs, us. When we shift, the lymph inside these semicircular canals, each ninety degrees to the other, sloshes like coffee in a cup on the rolling deck of a ship. The information collides with what we are told by our eyes and the soles of our feet, and we know, without needing to ask, the difference between a tilted head and a tilted body.

As time passes, the generative capacity we have to make our body anew fades. Our vision, our muscles, the feeling on the bottoms of our feet. The wobbles start small at first, then widen.

Our ear gets scarred like the rest of us. The minuscule stones that sit at the bottom of our ear and point to the ground, get shaken loose and tumble like gravel would in a moving tide. Instead of settling to the bottom, the loose stones stay high even when the water drops, and our brain is told that we are in two different places at the same time, and we can't believe what we're seeing. Turn this way if you want to stay straight, no this way, turn, turnturn. Our body lurches, our stomach too. We don't know where to fix our eyes, and they jitter from side to side. We close them. No place feels safe. There is no ease, no stillness. A physician, decades ago, who lost his sense of place described how he needed to wedge his head between two metal bars, so he could read without his heartbeat wiggling the letters.

Nothing works well for vertigo. More or less, you wait. Usually I'll prescribe medicines to mask the worst symptoms, dull the nausea a bit, sedate someone so they can sleep through the stress. Occasionally, activating all the contours of those canals in the ear, moving in every position and staying there until the symptoms fade, can ease the bad feeling. It's not clear whether this resets the gravel in the ear or our body learns to judge more accurately its new, tilted normal.

In most people, the problem resolves. The fluid starts to flow freely in the ear, shifts again to a natural resting place. Or the knowing thing that knows the middle accommodates the turbulence as noise that it mostly filters out. Dizziness becomes a new natural state.

Disequilibrium is a ruinous feeling if it lasts. When scientists want to study the effects of stress on animals, one of the ways to create it is to keep tilting a rat's cage in an unpredictable way. Slowly, surely, the rat loses weight, his immunity, develops ulcers, bleeds. Not being able to draw tight to the middle wears a system out. When one part is out of balance, it puts a greater load elsewhere.

At first, the middle is held so tightly, barely a quiver, but then we shake a bit. Our muscles fade. Our vision. Waver. More medicines to help us get from bed. Wobble. The process we are a part of is gathered less perfectly. Stumble. It wears through. Fall.

This past winter has been hard. My grandfather can't walk much anymore. He hasn't been able to go outside, and his muscles are disappearing, like his friends, family.

Many dark days, hours alone, heating up pancakes my mom left in the freezer.

He told me he's been to hospital a few times in the past month because of the dizziness. They take his blood pressure, do an electrocardiogram, draw blood. He's convinced that it is the withdrawn blood that makes him better, and tries to tell them to take more. But no one wants to listen to an old man.

W is for waiting.

The patient's head must have snapped backwards when he hit the ground. He slipped on a rag, or caught his boot, waved his arms once or twice but was unable to bring back balance, and spilled off the high scaffold. A split, silent second later, a wet thud, and a hardhat skittered across the cement floor.

I am looking at his CT scan. A thick vertebra sits perched a full centimetre ahead of the one below it, disrupting all three of the smooth curves I ask medical students to trace down the length of the cervical spine.

His spinal cord is cramped and bleeding, crushed about midway up his neck. An MRI would show the damage further. The hard rays from the CT scan light up the bone's calcium lattice but pass through softer things, like bleeding nerves, making them hard to see. Even without one, I know the injury is severe, that the cut must be complete.

He can feel nothing below his collarbones. If the swelling of the cord settles, he might be able to move his thumb a bit. This would be like receiving a key from jail, enough to allow him to control a chair, or a remote control, that small centimetre of cord and a flicker of a finger, the distance from staring at the ceiling to freedom.

He asked me if he would walk again. I told him it was too early to say.

A nurse at my shoulder studies the scan with me. I point out the damage. She nods.

"He wants to talk to you again."

"OK."

His chest is almost completely still. The nerves that control the ribs stop short of his brain now because of the break. His breathing is only from diaphragm, no more help from other muscles, and his belly balloons with each breath. If the swelling gets worse, it will cut off the brain's encouragement and he won't be able to breathe at all. He'll need a ventilator.

I stand at the head of his bed, lean over his face. His head is held in place by a thick, stiff collar. Tears push at the sides of his eyes.

"Hey, John."

"Doc."

"Yes."

". . ."

"John?"

"Please kill me."

"Oh, man. I can't."

Another day. I'm tired. Minor is busy. It's like that on Mondays. It's the only reliable predictor of volume. Over the weekend, either people suffer at home, not wanting to ruin a day off, or their family doctor picks up their frantic call after the weekend, sends them in. Waits are long.

". . . everyone else in the order they come."

A woman, an infection in her leg, red and swollen so wide it seemed to belong to a different person. We'd both stared at it, surprised.

"Doctorrrrr," she cried as I walked briskly past.

"I'll be back, ma'am," and I was, but not all of me, just my leaning body, one foot out the door. She asked me reasonable questions, she did, truly, but I told her, and myself, that I had no time for them, that she had taken too much from others already, and left her ballooned in bed, white sheet folded over her. Simon was waiting for handover, yeah that's it. I didn't want him to wait, not at this hour, so I left her there, told the nurses to discharge her, that I didn't want to speak to her again.

I slept in fits, and the next day, right after I woke, biked back to the fucking hospital, pulled her chart, phoned her up, sat there and listened to her ramblings until she was finished.

I'm back. The old words of Amharic feel natural on my tongue.

Aklilu, Biruk, and I deliver exams to the second class of emergency doctors. Finot, Gelaw, Gemechis, Demelesh, Tigist, Gelilah. I give them hard questions, try not to nod at the right answers. My poker face is strong as ever and they leave the room shaking their heads. In the dark basement of the learning centre, Biruk and I tally the final scores. They have all passed. Six more emergency doctors, ten total, one for every nine million now. Biruk is the only one of our first graduating class who is working in the ER. One has left the country, one can't find work. Haven't heard from the fourth for a while. No one knows how many lives she could save.

The group of teachers I brought from Toronto are divided into teams to cover different sides of Black Lion's ER. A half-dozen students in white coats lean in, trying to hear what one is saying about sick hearts and broken bones.

It's the end of the first day, and the other teacher stands in the middle of the floor, amazed. She sees me and walks over.

"Everyone is so sick."

I can only stay days now. At the end of the week, I will leave them behind, to learn and to teach.

When I board my plane back to Toronto on Friday, hundreds of doctors will be flying the other way to fight Ebola. In Canada, hospitals are pouring millions of dollars into a disease they'll not see. Up the hill from the tin ER, in those concrete-block residences, the cures lie in bed, staring at the ceiling, wishing they could have another chance with the imaginary pregnant woman hit by a car.

Back in the Toronto winter, I see John again in the ER, transferred from the hospice in which he lives. He has gained no use of this thumb. His arms are as thin as twigs, his lower legs just shin bone and shining skin.

He has a fever. I need to find where the infection is, because he can still feel nothing. A nurse helps me turn

him over. He smells of urine and baby powder. I peel
a bandage off his shoulder blade. Below it, raw flesh
that has worn through. Doesn't look infected. I do an
x-ray. It shows an early pneumonia. His blood pressure is very low.

"Think you'll need to come in for a couple of days."

"'Kay, Doc."

If he remembers me, it doesn't show.

I speak to my grandfather on the phone. His voice
quavers, his accent stronger every year. I apologize for
missing Christmas, tell him I'm coming home in the
summer, to spend some time with him again.

"Good, good," he says, hangs up.

In the learning centre, Aklilu shows me plans for a
new ER. "Two phases," he says, proudly. "First an
expansion, then a whole building."

I load my suitcase and a bicycle into the back of my
father's truck. We hug each other.

"See you soon, Dad."

I back out of the driveway and turn north.

My grandfather rises from the table.

He's so much older than I remember. How long have
I been gone?

"Fix yourself some lunch," he says. "Take whatever
you want." He sits back down. He can't stand.

I look through the fridge to make us some dinner. It
is mostly bare of fresh food. This is my parents' weekend
to visit. I told them I would do the shopping.

We talk. He is grateful for the company.

"You'd better catch a fish before it gets too dark,"
he says.

"You're right. I'll be back with a big one."

I walk to the lake. It is dusk, and the water is like oil. On it, loons call, then dive. They are new this summer, still learning their cry, how to hunt. The song comes out wrong, too shrill and too short. Or maybe they're saying something different than their parents.

Fish flies flutter in swarms towards grey-gold mounds of clouds a mile high. Dragonflies wrestle them, ruthless. One grabs a smaller version of herself in her claws, the same brilliant blue.

I take one of my cousin's rods from against the rowboat and call my brother in my headphones while I cast my hook, wind it back in. The lure is nearly home when out of the green blackness a pike shoots to the spoon. His long body twists as he snatches it and heads to the bottom.

Ziizzzzzzzz. My line rushes out.

"Do you want to call me back?" Dan says.

"No, no. It's OK."

Ziiiiizzzzzzz.

"Actually . . ."

He hangs up.

The fish starts to tire. I manoeuvre it down the dock, holding my rod far away from the posts so it can't wind around them, then skid him, flipping, onto the rocks.

He is about three feet, large enough to keep. I watch for a moment, branch in hand, as he tries to pull oxygen from the air, gills working like slow-beating wings, then crash the stick heavily on his flat brow. You must kill an animal right away, my grandpa taught me, or the fear gets into the meat. I call it adrenalin, but it's just a different name.

The last impulses of his bleeding brain ripple through his slick body, and his tail curls in twitches. I hit him a second time, and his red gills turns pale.

By the chokecherry tree, in the day's last light, I skin the fish on a grey wooden box. My grandfather's knives are all breathlessly sharp. I have not done this for years, never learned it well the first time, and when I finish, the skeleton has as much flesh on it as the fillets I've cut from its side.

I push the guts onto the grass and spray the box clean with a humming hose. I put the meat in a clear plastic bag, walk the guts and bones to the woodpile for the fox. In the kitchen window, my grandfather is sitting at the table, waiting.

XY is for a man.

He returns from the bathroom, his hair combed back, and shuffles slowly, holding on to the edge of a wall, then the counter, finally the kitchen chair. He smells of Aqua Velva aftershave. He is in his best clothes.

"We have time for a bit of lunch," I say. "At least a piece of sausage."

"I'll smell like garlic."

"The doctor won't mind."

He sits and waits. I pull a ring of kielbasa from the refrigerator, peel the plastic back, pull off a piece.

"Cucumber?"

"A little one."

We eat in silence. It is a bright blue day, still and hot.

A neighbour's truck is parked by the pin cherry tree. A man and a woman root through the strawberry patch.

"I don't know why I even planted a garden this year, Jim," he says, looking at the tall stalks of corn.

Yesterday, on my way up the hill, I stopped to pick peas, and the pods were bursting full, some already on the ground, overripe, no one to take them. My parents have their own.

"Did you see the deer?" he asks.

"This morning? Yeah. Two. Mom and daughter."

"I just saw the doe. If I could have opened the door, I would have put a BB into her. She can eat someone else's garden."

I asked him yesterday if he wanted to go to the trapline after the doctor, to check the wild rice. No, no, he said, we'd need a chainsaw, and you don't know how to use it. Instead, he let me cut the grass, but only after he took a turn on the tractor to show me how.

"How's the pipe under the road?" he asks. "Still holding?"

"Seems to be," I say.

A hole burst in a black plastic pipe that pumped water from the lake. A puddle formed where it ran under the road, and the pump was whining nonstop to keep up the pressure. It would burn out.

The filling end was held fast to the bottom of the lake by two plates of metal, twenty metres from shore, too heavy for a single man to lift. Maybe I could drag it, though.

"You can't do it, Jim."

"I could try."

"No, no. I'll get Zenny."

His neighbour, with a buzzing boat, tugged the weighted end closer to shore, the slack allowing us to pull the leaking section from the sand. A rupture the size of a pencil lead sprayed water. Zenny and I talked about how best to cut free the burst section, then rejoin it.

"Just get a clamp and a piece of inner tube. It will never leak," Grandpa said, and took off up the hill, side-saddle on the quad. Zenny and I were left behind to argue different ideas. "Hey . . . look," I said, pointing to the pipe. A half-dozen clamps holding pieces of inner tube, some rusted, years old, all of them dry.

"Pull the car up," Grandpa says now, leaning on the rail at the bottom of the steps. He won't take my arm. I back it up from the garage and open the passenger door. He takes a teetering step in between the railing and the car, grabs the frame, painfully lowers himself in. We back up to the silver metal tank, full of gasoline, next to the freezing house, where fish could be kept cool.

They used to haul slabs of ice, five hundred pounds each, to it. It would take four men, one horse, and a day to get ice to the freezer. If you were smart, he told me, you built the platform leading to the freezer at a particular angle, so you could slide the ice slowly, without it picking up speed. More than one hand had lost fingers.

One day, the ice company bought an electric saw. You could cut the ice into blocks and slide them with a pick into a truck. He could do it alone.

I finish fuelling.

"The gas tank," he says, pointing. "Check how full." I tap along the metal, trying to listen for the point where the vibrations narrow because of the fluid interface behind it, like I would on a person's back, tapping for a lung full of pus. The whole drum rings like a bell. I can detect no change.

"No, no," he says, frustrated, tries to get out of the car before giving up. "Hold the nozzle upright near the top of the tank, and open it. That's right. Move it slowly down. Slower." About halfway down the tank, gas burbles over my hand.

"Good. Half. Let's go."

People coast down the hill at night and steal gas from him. "You should put a lock on it," I say, putting the car into drive.

No, if people want to steal, they will just break it. The only thing he locks are his guns.

The small town near where he lives is quiet today. Alberta's short summer is almost over, and everyone is on the lake. We park at the entrance to the doctor's office, and he moves slowly up the ramp, holding on to the rail, and opens the door.

"I'm Mike Maskalyk."

"Right this way, Mr. Maskalyk." A woman leads us into a cold, bright room. "The doctor will be right with you."

My grandfather waits, his hands in his lap, quiet. We are here for me, not for him. I called a few weeks ago, to make sure he and I could come in together. It's the one thing he'll still let me do.

Yesterday we sat, and made a list of what bothered him most.

"My knees, Jim. I can't stand." And the dizziness. Cataracts too.

"I'm going to take the first five minutes to talk about what you told me in doctors' language, OK?"

"All right."

The doctor comes in, not quite thirty. He's from Saskatchewan, in his last two weeks of training. I congratulate him.

"Now, I make it a habit of not doctoring people I love, but I want to explain some things."

"Um, OK," the young doctor says, looking at my grandfather.

"First, understand. My grandfather, under no circumstances, wants to leave his home. Everything we do is going to be an attempt to keep him there, with as much freedom as possible. The greatest risk he has is falling."

I keep talking. He writes as fast as he can, asks a few questions of my grandfather, then stands, opens the door, and points us down the hall. My grandfather waves my hand away.

A nurse meets us, puts a cuff on his upper arm, measures his pressure, asks him to sit down. They talk cucumbers. She takes his pressure again. It is almost 15 points lower when he's standing. Could be that his brain isn't getting enough flow when he changes position, making him dizzy. Back in the cold room, the doctor suggests cutting the dose of a pill in half, arranging a home monitor for his heart.

"Sure, sure," my grandfather says as the nurse tells him of an appointment in a few weeks, and he shuffles past, without looking up.

At home, I cut the pills in two. A split tablet skitters across the table and falls to the floor.

"Do you want some iced tea?"

"Half a cup," he says.

I go to the fridge, find the glass carafe.

"When are you going to settle down?" he asks.

"Soon."

"You're like my brother Bill. He could never sit still, not for five minutes. One day he drove here all the way from California, said he was going to stay a week and help me fish, but by the next day, he was packed up again. Nervous."

I nod.

Here it goes.

"Do you miss Grandma?"

"Sometimes."

"What about Uncle Miles?"

"That was a sad thing, Jim. He used to be here every day."

"Do you think about that much?"

"Not much. What's the use?"

He looks out the window. The hummingbird feeder is full with sweet water. Every few minutes, one hovers, dips his long beak into the fake yellow flower, drinks. Wasps curl under the bottoms, licking drips.

"It's good Mom and Dad come here so much," I say after a time. Every second weekend, even in the blowing snow. They work from the moment they arrive until the moment they leave. The weekends between, they take care of their own land.

"Oh, they've been real good. Real good."

His glass is empty. The clock ticks behind us.

I pull my phone from my pocket, put it on the table. He looks at it.

"Those things are just terrible. Some people come over, and they're just staring at it. You can't even talk."

"You should see the city. People walk down the streets looking at them the whole time. They'd make bad hunters."

"No good at all. Those phones are the worst thing ever been invented. I remember . . ."

Snowshoes. Dogsleds. Teams of horses. The first cars. Breaking his knee carrying a beaver on his back. Falling through the ice. Losing his way in the blinding snow. Months alone, far away from another human soul.

The youngest of eleven, the oldest two born in the Ukraine, him in Alberta, near the trapline. The family came off the boat with their clothes, a scythe, a whetstone, ready to farm, and found a place filled with trees. His father died when he was eight. Then a brother, a sister. TB. Measles. They are all dead now.

His older brothers didn't go to school. There was none close, and with no father, they were too busy. When spring came, they planted crops on land they had cleared, and killed deer. At the first frost, they harvested, started shooting moose, then trapped and skinned through long winter nights until spring came again.

My grandfather was young when a school was built nearby. He went through Grade 8. It was as far as you could go. In his final year, the teacher asked the boys what they were going to be when they grew up. Farmer, farmer, farmer, farmer, each one said in turn, because it was all they knew. The teacher came to my grandfather.

I can't say, he answered, knowing only that a farmer was the only thing he *didn't* want to be. The teacher walked back behind his long wood desk, ripped a piece of paper in two, wrote on each half, and put his hands behind his back.

Pick one, he said to my grandfather.

He chose.

Hunter, it read.

"What was in the other?" I ask.

"Trapper."

One day, after class, he waded through the snow to check his snares. He saw the prints of a coyote, then heard it struggling. The loop had caught its leg instead of its airway. He took a dead branch and approached, but the animal heard him and tore more viciously. The willow was bent to the ground, the wire starting to slide off. As he got close, it slipped loose. The coyote turned to my grandfather, snarling.

"Did you run?"

"No. I jumped on it."

He was bitten on the leg, but killed the coyote with a knife, then limped home, the animal across his shoulders. It was worth two bucks. There was no choice.

The stories keep tumbling. My grandfather passed a friend who owned the first vehicle in the area, walking along the long road to the nearest mailbox, and asked him why he didn't drive his shiny new truck. The man started in surprise. I forgot I had one, he said. Call for moose once, maybe twice, and then just sit, wait for the crashes of the horns to grow closer.

I've never heard him talk this much. I listen, rapt. Some of the stories I've heard before, some are new. It doesn't matter.

"What is it like, to be old?"

"No good."

"Why not?"

"I can't do anything I used to love, Jim."

"Like what?"

"Skinning muskrats. I could do it all night. Beavers, coyotes I never liked. But muskrats, I just loved them. They're so clean. Such beautiful animals."

"Are you afraid of dying?"

"No."

His hands are thick, bunched at the knuckles, covered in spots and scars. He looks me in the eye, holds my gaze, raises a trembling finger.

"When it's my time, you let me go. If I can't go to the bathroom or take care of myself, that's it."

I nod.

"I don't want to be in no hospital. No tubes. None."

"OK . . . Grandpa?"

"What?"

"Why won't you take my arm?"

He swivels his chair towards the window, puts his hand on the table. Two hummingbirds are duelling. They hover, dart. Their throats are red.

I should know the answer. This is his story, and, once he starts, he'll never stop.

"Do you want to go to the trapline?" I ask again, glancing at the clock.

"It's too late, Jim. I'll get someone to take me next week. Dylan or Kayne. They know about rice."

"All right."

He thinks for a second. "Maybe you can drive me to the big island. To see the water."

Over the lakes, their smooth surface puckered by fish, a causeway connects a large island to the shore.

"Slow down and drive real close to the rail," he says, and peers through the window.

"This road used to be a sandbar. We couldn't cross it, and to fish this part of the lake"—he points to his side—"we would need to take the boat all the around the island. It would take over an hour, so one day, me and another fisherman hired a team of horses and one of those scrapers, you know, what they used to build roads before machines?"

I don't know, but nod.

"We hauled the sand, about ten feet or so, until it was deep enough that we could pole the boat across. We still had to lift the motor, but it saved us a long time. When we came to set nets next, the water was flowing from this part of the lake"—he gestures again—"to this side, like a river. It was a current. So when I heard they were going to build this causeway, I went to one of those meetings, you know, with the town, and told them. They said they would blast out a space for the water to flow, but they never did, they just blocked it. Now look." He waved a hand at the thick fields of weeds that spread away from the road on both sides.

We drive on, and the trees stretch high around the road. Once, you could only take a boat here. We pass people on bikes. A man scowls at our dust. The forest thins and the lake glints through.

A sign saying Viewpoint points to a wooden bridge, a platform beyond. I slow to a stop.

"You want to go see?"

"No. You go."

"Are you sure?"

"I'm sure."

I turn the car off, climb out. Leaves flutter. A crow lifts off the ground. I step onto the wooden slats, and the ground falls away before me. On the lake, a set of smaller islands, festooned with gulls, cormorants. I hear the cacophony of their calls. In the car, my grandfather sits alone, hidden behind the glass and the sun's reflection.

Z is for ze end.

In a farmer's field, last year's grass, rolled and heaped, frosted with snow. On the side of the stack, spray-painted in green script fifteen feet high, "$20 hay, $10 straw."

The road was once busy with machines hauling other machines north towards oil, or south for repair. Not these days. Ice piles in the middle of my lane, and I pass only a few vehicles. Closer to Edmonton, I saw empty fields of trailers that once held thousands of working men.

I am driving to my grandfather's house. I spent last night in the home where I was born. I know every light switch in the dark, each step that creaks. It was quiet. My parents are already at the lake. My brother is on his way.

The bare trees blur by and I'm lost between the landscape's white palette and thoughts on the end.

I watched a friend die. Though we didn't know each other long, she cared for me like a son, helped me keep my home clean for next to nothing until she got cancer. A surgeon cut off one breast, then another, but it had already moved from there. A cell travelled to her brain, made millions more that didn't belong. She gave up quickly with this news. Some people do that.

She was afraid and alone. I spoke with her daughter, a continent away, on a crackling connection. We were never close, she said. In a few short weeks, my friend was moved from her basement apartment to the nearest hospital, an hour's bike ride from my home, a distance she had travelled by bus twice a month, all of her cleaning supplies bundled in a tartan sack.

The first day I visited, she was sitting up in bed, eating ice cream. I had never seen her outside of my apartment.

Are you afraid?

A little, Dr. James.

A week later, she was in a morphine dream. I touched her hand. Her eyes fluttered open. "Dr. James? Is that you? Am I in heaven?"

"Not yet."

Her eyes blinked closed.

My final time, I sat on a bench outside the hospital. I paid hard attention to the ends of things, sounds, thoughts, sensations, like my teacher had taught me.

I took the elevator up to her room. She was unconscious. Her breath came in hitches. I squeezed her hand, and her brow furrowed for a second, then smoothed.

I stood beside her, watching. She was coming apart.

Shakeshakeshake. The vibrations kept moving faster and faster, then slowed, then stopped.

I pass by Smoky Lake, the town between the trapline and the farm. Too far from oil or city, it has been left out of the boom, and its rim of houses haven't changed. Farmer. Farmer. Farmer.

Jack pine lines the ditches in tall stands. A break. A field. Kikino Métis settlement. Our trapline starts just behind.

Last time I was there, I drove to it alone, got lost a few times on the way to the cabin. Dan told me a bear had torn apart the outhouse, and sure enough, there it stood, its plywood door in two pieces, the roof ripped off.

I walked down the same cutline where I shot that moose. It was late summer, and the grass was high. Mosquitoes buzzed at my neck. The bitter taste of repellent mixed with sweat stung the tip of my tongue.

At the bottom of the hill, where my brother had knelt and stuck a knife through the hot fur of the moose I had shot, a hundred straight goldenrod stalks shot to the sun. In the moose-sized patch of grass, green bugs hopped stem to stem, moths fluttered, making families.

Endings, beginnings, who can tell?

A familiar curve, and a sign for a place where my mom went to school near her farm. An echo of a feeling from when I was a boy, an excitement that soon I would be at my favourite place.

A final turn, and I'm rolling down the frozen drive towards his house. My brother's minivan is outside the door, Adrienne, his wife, pulling shut its wide side. She turns at the crunch of my tires, smiles and waves. I pull up in front of the freezer house, alongside my parents' white car.

I bang the snow from my boots and open the door. The floor is festooned with shoes of all sizes, black Bouvier dogs, and bags of books.

"Have you guys been here for a month?" I say to my brother, standing at the top of the stairs to the basement and my bed by the furnace.

"About five minutes."

We smile at each other. He hugs me hard.

My mom peers around the corner, smiling, kisses me on the cheek.

"Your dad's outside. Something about the electricity to the trailer."

"OK."

I go through to the living room. Through the large front window, the lake is criss-crossed with cleated snowmobile tracks. The bones of a dock pulled to shore, my parents' trailer beside it. My dad pulls a power cord through a deep drift. Beyond him are a few ice-fishing huts.

Adrienne is pulling on Sam's snowmobile pants. He whispers, "Mom, can we stay an extra day?" I laugh. That sentence was mine for so many years.

"How's . . . Jim?" and my grandfather turns from the silent TV.

"I'm good, Grandpa. Glad to be here."

"I think Sam and Lucy are getting ready to go fishing."

"Guess I'd better get ready too."

The wind is biting. If I close my eyes for more than a second, ice sticks my lashes together, and the blink pulls at the roots.

My brother pushes the auger all the way down to its bleating engine, and water sputters onto the snow. The ice is more than a metre thick. We borrowed the machine from our aunt. My grandpa's has gone missing.

Sam and my niece, Lucy, dangle their clear threads into the holes, neither sure what to do if they get a bite.

The sun breaks through a few minutes before it sets, and casts long shadows onto orange snow, then dips below the trees. The temperature falls, and the wind picks up. The kids can no longer see their frozen bait below them.

"All right, dinnertime. Back in the sled." Dan and I take off in separate snowmobiles towards home, the kids bouncing behind us, hands over their ears from the noise.

We eat as a family, my parents older, greyer, my dad limping a bit, my mother too. The kids eat on their knees at the coffee table, chatting softly. At the end of the table, my grandfather sits, saying only, "Pass the salt . . . the bread . . ."

The conversation grows louder with wine. I watch him. He has only water. Whenever someone speaks, he looks them in the eye until they are done. There is nothing nervous about him.

He goes to bed early. Dan and Adrienne put the kids to sleep on the floor, then stand over the kitchen sink, doing the dishes. My parents are on the couch, remembering. Talk turns to people they've said goodbye to, some of whom I know. I tell them my last wishes, should they ever need to know them. If I can't laugh, or show love, let me go. Me too, my mom says. I don't think about it much, says my dad.

The next day, it's time for everyone to go. Slowly coats and keys are pulled towards the door, then into cars.

"Bye . . . bye . . . so nice . . . love you . . . you too . . ."

I am staying. He needs someone to drive him to the lawyer, make some last arrangements for the will.

We play crib. I lose badly. I cook some moose my mother thawed. We talk about the end. I want to make it beautiful.

"I just don't want any fighting."

"OK."

"That's it. And everything is fair."

"I understand."

The next morning, before we drive into town, my cousin comes over. My grandfather tells us about 50-cent pieces my grandmother had collected for years. They're in the basement, he tells me, in a trunk by the stairs.

"I want to go down."

My cousin above, me below, we watch him on the steep stairs, as he painfully puts down one foot, then the other, until he's on the cracked cement floor, furnace roaring by my bed, antlers and bullets beside it, a picture of him as a young man, cigarette in his fingers, coyotes all around.

"I haven't been down here for two years," he says, squeaking a chair in front of a metal chest. "Open it."

Dylan does. On the top section, folders of photos. There's my grandfather, in Banff, when the town was just a few houses big. My uncle's high school diploma. A picture of my dad, Sam's age, same shy smile. Dylan and I pass them back and forth.

"Who's this? . . . And this . . . you?"

A picture of four children, dirty faces, about a hundred years ago. My grandpa nods, looks at the photo briefly, then hands it back.

"No coins?"

"Not so far."

We pull off the top shelf. Stacks of tablecloths, napkins. Must and mothballs.

"Doesn't look like they're here," I say, and I rummage deeper, finding only fabric.

My hand hits a metal can.

I pull off the top layers, and find four brown tobacco tins, coins sliding back and forth inside them. The first few are full of quarters and nickels, half-rolled for the bank. The fourth I open to a list describing all the rare coins it holds. Half-dollars, old pennies.

We divide these into four, one for each grandson, write our names on pieces of paper, and put them in plastic Ziploc bags, then help him back up the stairs.

The next morning, I sit with a lawyer who draws out Grandpa's simple request as close to an hour as he can make it, then we walk on the snowy sidewalk towards his car, him leaning heavily between his cane and a brown picket fence.

I stop and buy him some final things. A plastic jar of nuts, strawberry jam, on special. Lunch meat. The square kind, he says, with the rind. The boy working the deli and I puzzle over the cylinders of pressed meat until we find it. I take the lake road home.

We are at his table, my car idling.

He fixes me with his bright green eyes. They don't quiver.

"Are you happy with my will?"

"Yes."

Is it OK for me to let go?

It's OK.

Life isn't just one big funeral, you know, Jim.

It isn't?

No. It's full of living too, and for that, you don't have to wait. Do you get it now?

ACKNOWLEDGEMENTS.

I have written above the desk where I wrote many of these pages, "This is a book about relationships . . . from our cells to our body, our body to our friends and family, them to strangers and people far away, even all living things." It pleases me to think that connections matter, that they repeat in similar patterns all the way down.

As such, this is not mine alone, though its words are. If, through them, I have done anyone an injustice, at least one is failing to properly capture how valuable they have been in my life, and to the world.

First, and most deeply, I am indebted to Clare Pain, the architect of the abiding relationship between Toronto and Addis Ababa, whose natural generosity is so large, that it included not just me, but dozens of other teachers.

Her assurance that change, with the right intention, however incremental, is inevitable, has helped me understand that it is the action, not the outcome, that matters most.

There would be no opportunity for such action if it weren't for the determination of my many Ethiopian friends. You hold the space open, both that room and your hearts, against great odds, with your kindness and commitment. I offer my lifelong support, and am excited to watch the next years both from afar and beside you. It saddens me that I have only been able to include a few of your names. To capture the true worth of your attention, not on emergency medicine, but creating a better future for us all, would require another book. That one, though, is yours to write. Perhaps I can be in it. I'm hoping if my character can be a kind of swashbuckling mercenary who has changed his ways, but it's up to you.

To my many teachers, in the hospital and outside, who helped me understand that if I didn't offer myself the same care I was expected to provide to others, I would never get it right. To Jane Lemaire for teaching me to get out of the body's way, to Massey Beveridge, who helped me understand that medicine was social and political, and to Gabor Maté for extolling me to look ever deeper. To Shinzen Young, many deep bows for both my practice and for your tireless pointing. To Viola Fodor, for leading me to the difference between will and willpower, for your encouragement to know myself more deeply with faith that I would love what I found, and most of all for offering me the same question again and again until I understood what you were asking: "So. How are you?"

To my colleagues at St. Michael's Hospital. Thank

you for giving me a place that is as close as I can get to MSF in Toronto. Your work is endless, too often thankless, but you show up every day, and teach me how laugh. I show up every day because of you. To the many clinicians and scholars at the University of Toronto, particularly Megan Landes and Cheryl Hunchak, who have, since the beginning, held the direction for a community of doctors, my admiration and solidarity.

To my patients, my greatest guides, I am grateful for your trust, and for the daily opportunity to deserve it. You show me, in Ethiopia as in Toronto, that the healing space that emerges with true human connection depends neither on privilege nor geography. Many of you have informed the people I describe in these pages, but I have changed details to protect your privacy, not just your sicknesses or worries, but age, sex, country.

To Bruce Westwood for encouraging this book by reminding me that getting it wrong while struggling to get it right was part of the process. To Martha Kanya-Forstner, my editor and favourite reader. You helped me tame a nearly impossible work into something simple that I believe in. As any writer knows, there can be no greater gift.

To Jeff Warren, my friend and fellow Consciousness Explorer, thanks for being such an enthusiastic person to both meditate and write beside, for dragging me to the library, while convincing me that three hours of writing per day was the most anyone could hope for. To Mark, Greg, Matt, Ian, Michael, my friends, through it all. To Grace, for your kindness and wisdom.

My father, Milton, my mother, Lucille, my brother, Dan. Adrienne, Sam, Lucy. Your unconditional love is what inspires mine to impossible heights. Though I don't see you as often as I would like, you are with me every day, for I set it as my goal in the hospital to treat strangers as gently as I would you.

Last, my grandfather, Michael. I was hunting a week ago (my brother shot a doe, I missed a moose), and came up the cutline from Partridge Corner to find an idling truck. The driver was a man who, when he was a young boy, on a Christmas after his mother and sister both died, you delivered a sack of toys to, a bigger one than you gave your own children. You were in the passenger seat. All week long my mom told me how you were hoping to find a way to the trapline, to see us, telling her, "I just want to be a part of it, and there you were, in the passenger seat." You rolled down the window, and we talked about the tracks you had seen on the road, the wolves I had heard, and as I was about to pull away, you leaned over and touched my hand.

You're part of it, and part of me. Thank you for being the man you are, and showing me that knowing how to be a man, alone with yourself at the end of your life, is the same as knowing it now.

Should you be keen on following this story to its never-end, visit jamesmaskalyk.com and follow the doors. You'll see, already, in the short time since this book ended in Ethiopia, there is adenosine and antropine, there are ventilators in the ER, and that some of the young doctors, once wide-eyed and new, know both the ABC's and the principle of "sickest first" well enough to pass them to other capable hands.

ABOUT THE AUTHOR

JAMES MASKALYK, bestselling author of the critically acclaimed *Six Months in Sudan*, is an emergency-room physician, award-winning teacher, and member of Médecins Sans Frontières. He teaches meditation with the Consciousness Explorers Club and currently divides his time between Toronto and Addis Ababa.

A NOTE ABOUT THE TYPE

Life on the Ground Floor has been set in Sabon, an "old style" serif originally designed by Jan Tschichold in the 1960s.

The roman is based on types by Claude Garamond (c.1480– 1561), primarily from a specimen printed by the German printer Konrad Berner. (Berner had married the widow of fellow printer Jacques Sabon, hence the face's name.)